natural
woman

Other titles by Penelope Sach

Detox
The Healing Effects of Herbal Tea
Take Care of Yourself
The Little Book of Wellbeing
Natural Health for Men

natural
woman

PENELOPE
SACH

Frog, Ltd.
Berkeley, California

Published by Frog, Ltd.

Frog, Ltd. books are distributed by
North Atlantic Books
P.O. Box 12327
Berkeley, California 94712
www.northatlanticbooks.com

First published by Penguin Books Australia Ltd. 2002

Book design by Susannah Low, Penguin Design Studio
Author photograph by Louise Lister

Printed in Canada

This book is not intended to replace or supersede professional medical advice. Neither the author nor the publisher may be held responsible for claims arising from the mistaken identity of any herbs or the inappropriate use of any remedy or healing regime contained in this book.

Library of Congress Cataloging-in-Publication Data

Sach, Penelope.
    Natural woman: how to beat fatigue, look radiant, and take control of your health / by Penelope Sach.
        p. cm.
    Includes Index.
    Reprint. Previously printed by Penguin in Australia in 2002.
    ISBN 1-58394-091-X (pbk.)
    1. Women--Health and hygiene. 2. Self-care, Health. 3. Alternative medicine. I. Title.

RA778.S179 2003
613'.04244--dc22

2003017346

1 2 3 4 5 6 7 8 9 TRANSCON 08 07 06 05 04 03

Contents

To my mother and sister

Introduction

WOMEN ARE TRULY REMARKABLE. They nurture, they love, they work, they play, they bear children, and they are forever trying to balance their lives with the responsibilities of partners, family, work, and friends. Combine the stresses of work, children, and partners with the issues of health and aging, and the modern woman has much to contend with. Women now have a much longer life expectancy, and so the major issues of sustained good health and aging gracefully have become a priority. The advertising for many cosmetic companies promises wonders but delivers very little. Why? Because the greater life forces are really to do with good nutrition, stress management, and high self-esteem. And those are the forces that we deal with throughout this book.

The women I have treated over the years—many of whom never thought they could possibly achieve great vitality, happiness, and balance—are a walking example that anything is possible with a little discipline, motivation, and organization.

Self-esteem is essential for women. When a woman loses her self-esteem, it impacts on her entire life—not only her health and vitality but also her decision-making abilities, relationships, confidence, career, and her inner consciousness. Improving self-esteem takes courage, lots of soul-searching, and determination. But women are great at this, aren't they? They have a superb ability, once they are motivated, to really change.

As a healer I have observed women regain their self-esteem through improving their physical health. This, in turn, improves their mental health. I often say to my clients, "Change your eating habits, include exercise, and do something spiritual for yourself and then see what is left over." Rarely do they have to spend money on long-term counselling. The world opens up to them when they open up to it with gradual changes. Habits are difficult to break but you can reap great rewards.

Natural medicine seems to have a particular significance for women. Traditionally, it was very much part of a woman's domain. Throughout the centuries in many cultures women held a vital relationship with the earth. They were the gatherers of the seeds, nuts, berries, and herbs needed for both food and medicines. The knowledge they gleaned has been passed down through the ages in legends, recipes and, of course, "old wives' tales," many of which have their basis in truth. It's only in the last decade that scientists are proving with modern methods the profound therapeutic effects of many plants and herbs. For example, black cohosh has lately been found to have powerful properties and can effectively treat menopausal symptoms. This was a plant well known to the American Indians, who used it for this purpose. Similarly chasteberry (*Vitex agnus-castus*), which was mentioned in the records of Hippocrates in the fourth century B.C., is today recognized by the regulating health body of the German government as an effective treatment for abnormal menstrual cycles and pre-menstrual tension (PMT).

It seems only natural to turn to these and other natural therapies as an aid to dealing with modern life. Each chapter in this book focuses on one or more of the most common issues faced by women today and offers natural preventative and treatment regimes.

The ten most commonly asked questions I hear in my practice are:

- How can I have more energy?
- How can I get to sleep and stop feeling tired?
- How can I lose weight?
- How can I have a flat stomach?
- How can I find time to exercise?
- How can I improve my skin?
- How can I have sparkling eyes and clear whites?
- How can I make my nails stronger?
- How can I improve my libido?
- How can I improve my memory?

The information in this book will answer all these questions, and more. This book is about getting on top of your life and making the changes necessary to improve your quality of life.

Where possible, I incorporate programs for specific areas of your health following the formulae I use for my individual clients. This includes daily practices you can use to prevent the problems occurring—problems such as weight gain, hormonal imbalance, poor skin, hair and nails, depression, and anxiety. Each chapter will offer you solutions. Use this advice first if you are already suffering a problem. If you are not ready for all the information in the problem area and you cannot face taking all the medicines and vitamins suggested, then begin with the first supplement only. Lead on to the second supplement when you feel ready. Once the condition has improved, you should consult the vital living program (see chapter 11) and incorporate it into your lifestyle, or you may prefer to begin the program first to see the effect it has on your overall health.

Adopt the principles in this book and see for yourself that renewed vitality and healthy ways lead to better quality of life. Take up that study you have always wanted to do. Renew old friendships you once cherished. Speak to the man you always admired and tell him so. Take that holiday you always wanted, even if it is for a shorter time than you wished. Change your job if it's really not for you and try something different. Incorporate simple pleasures into your life.

This book is all about women. In the seventeen years I have been working with natural medicines in my private practice, I have seen thousands of women. In most cases, they have been able to improve their quality of life and their physical and mental outlook by using the sort of advice I have written down in this book.

May you too experience a new lease of life.

1

A woman's appearance

EVERY WOMAN I see as a client usually mentions her skin, hair, and nails. Often she complains of dull, tired skin, dry hair, and brittle breaking nails. The women prone to these problems are often busy women and mothers who don't have a regular, balanced diet. They may be vegetarian and not getting sufficient protein from legumes or they may eat sporadically, not eating lunch or just having a salad with no protein component.

The following are major factors in maintaining beautiful skin, hair, and nails:

- protein
- calcium

- high fluid intake
- good digestion
- hormonal balance.

Protein

Skin, hair, and nails are all high in protein. To regenerate skin tissue, hair follicles, and nail beds, a woman's diet must include plenty of protein.

Every day you should include at least two proteins from the following:

- fish
- chicken
- red meat
- legumes (soya beans, lima beans, adzuki beans, lentils)
- nuts (almonds are excellent and also sesame seeds and pumpkin seeds)
- eggs (two eggs—or egg whites for those with high cholesterol—every second day)
- cheese
- rice, soya, or dairy milk
- yogurt (a mild source of protein).

Note: Drink soya, rice, or low-fat milk in between meals or as a protein meal in the mornings. Add yogurt and blended fruit for a more filling meal.

Calcium

Calcium is essential for skin, hair, and nails. If you have eliminated dairy foods from your diet, then a supplement is advisable. Eating a small tub of yogurt daily is a sure way to obtain calcium. Make sure it contains acidophilus, the friendly bacteria that assists digestion. Low-fat milk or soya milk with added calcium or low-fat white cheese are also good sources of calcium and should be included in the diet daily. However, fermented cheeses such as blue vein and cheddar can disturb the digestion; avoid them, especially if you are prone to a bloated stomach.

Calcium is found in almonds and sesame seeds, which make good snacks or can be ground and added to cereal or low-fat milkshakes. The small bones of tinned fish like salmon and sardines are also a good source of calcium as are parsley, watercress, spinach, and onions.

High fluid intake

A high fluid intake promotes good circulation, which is vital to the health of skin, hair, and nails. Eight glasses of pure water or herbal tea per day keep the nutrients flowing through the blood and clear the waste from the cell tissues. Water assists the liver and kidneys to remove toxins from the body. Many of my clients have increased their fluid consumption to eight glasses a day and their skin has become much clearer and fresher.

In the morning, I highly recommend a glass of water with the juice of half a lemon, which acts as a mini-detox for the liver.

Good digestion

Chew slowly and sit down to eat any food. Protein is broken down by the acids of the stomach, so a rushed meal encourages poor protein metabolism and bloating (see pages 37–42).

Hormonal balance

Fluctuations in hormonal balance during pregnancy and menopause often affect a woman's appearance. Dry skin, hair loss, and brittle nails often occur when women have just had a baby, or when their cycles have stopped for a while due to stress or heavy exercise. It can happen when a woman is breastfeeding but not eating enough protein and calcium. Many women experiencing menopause also find their skin becomes dry and their hair and nails tend to be brittle. This is due to a drop in progesterone and oestrogen that occurs at this stage. To counteract these problems, include two teaspoonfuls of flaxseed oil in your diet daily. Follow the vital living program (see chapter 11), and refer also to chapter 6 for the specific hormonal issues.

Radiant skin

❧ Exclude all fried foods, cordials, and carbonated drinks.

❧ Cut out all white sugar. Use a little honey or brown sugar as a sweetener if you need it.

❧ Eat cold-water fish such as salmon, mackerel, or tuna three times a week.

❧ Include a raw carrot juice daily for the natural vitamin A content, which helps to regenerate skin cells.

❧ Alcohol and caffeine are very dehydrating for the skin. Try to avoid them for a least six weeks and then include only a few cups/glasses twice a week. When you reintroduce coffee into your diet, limit yourself to one a day followed by a large glass of filtered water or herbal tea to cleanse the kidneys.

❧ Try Campari and soda during summer, as this is less dehydrating than wine and champagne. You may even like to cut back on wine by drinking a little gin and tonic or vodka instead. Avoid cocktails as they are loaded with sugar and will upset the acid and alkaline balance of your skin.

❧ For nursing mothers, after the baby is weaned, take two evening primrose oil capsules daily to bring radiance back to your skin. This can also help you to regain regular periods.

To combat dry skin include the following supplements in your diet:
- Evening primrose oil: two capsules each morning and night.

- An antioxidant supplement with vitamins A, E, and C: two each morning after breakfast.

Acne

This can be a major problem for teenagers during puberty and adults with a poor diet and/or patterns of acne in their family history. Hormones are also the main cause of acne in women. For teenage girls, acne can be the most embarrassing and depressing part of growing up. At this age hormones are becoming active and can cause radical changes to moods and skin. Increased oestrogen can clog up the liver pathways, which need natural treatments and natural antibiotic cleansers to try and keep them clear.

Treatment

❦ One tablet of chasteberry each morning. This herb will help to balance and regulate hormonal cycles, particularly in teenage girls.

❧ Two garlic oil capsules daily, which will assist in keeping the blood clear of impurities from the liver.

❧ One teaspoonful of echinacea liquid, which acts as a natural antibiotic, daily.

❧ Check your iron and B_{12} levels with your doctor, especially if you're vegetarian, as an iron deficiency could contribute to bad skin.

❧ A drug called Retin A can be prescribed for severe cases of acne. This drug can have quite severe side effects on the liver, so you need to discuss these with your doctor. Generally you must have regular liver checks when on the medication. I often give a liver detox tonic to clients on Retin A, to take the overload off the liver. This can be taken in conjunction with the medication and also with garlic supplements and vitamin B. The tonic consists of equal parts of dandelion, schisandra, artichoke and St Mary's thistle and a flavoring of licorice or peppermint. Take one teaspoonful two to three times a day during the time of medication and for two months after. If you don't want to take this during the medication, take it after the Retin A course to help maintain the complexion and detox the liver.

Nutrition for teenage girls

- Cut out as many fatty foods as possible (to take the overload off the liver) and include a fresh orange juice and a fresh carrot juice daily.
- Cut back on red meats (two to three times a week) and include fish such as salmon and tuna.
- Cut back on carbonated drinks and use fresh water and fresh juices instead.
- If you like only two or three vegetables, concentrate on eating these daily. (For parents, it is better to work with your teenager than against her, as moods can vary considerably during adolescence.)
- If you are playing heavy sport at school, include one complex vitamin B per day for energy and clearing the liver at a faster rate.

Eczema

Generally, the yeast in bread, cheese, wine, and vinegar adds to the aggravation of eczema, as do all acidic foods (including orange juice, strawberries, and passionfruit), refined sugar, and chocolate. A doctor can diagnose any specific food allergies, but reducing your intake of these foods should help this skin condition. Cut out or avoid all foods to which you are sensitive or allergic.

If your symptoms worsen at particular times of the year, traditionally during spring or autumn, start your treatment three weeks before the expected onset. Travelling to drier climates or countries can also be a catalyst for eczema.

Treatment

🌺 In very severe cases, use prescription cortisone cream
(1 percent) to get the eczema under control quickly
and then try natural remedies, which include applying
calendula cream and sorbolene cream with vitamin E daily.

❧ After an initial outbreak, for the first four days take three capsules of omega–3 and –6 oils after each meal, then as the skin improves you may lower the dosage to a preventative dose of two capsules both morning and night. In summer, you can lower the dose to two capsules per day.

❧ Fill a muslin bag with oats and add it to a warm bath. It will soothe and calm the skin. Apply sorbolene cream afterwards.

❧ If scratching the eczema has caused bleeding, take an echinacea tablet three times a day to assist the immune system and also a garlic tablet three times a day for its antibacterial properties. If the bleeding is severe, you may need a prescribed antibiotic to get the rash under control and then use the naturopathic treatment measures.

❧ Take two evening primrose oil capsules three times a day until improvement and then lower the dose as improvement continues.

❀ Take a tonic made from equal parts of red clover, dandelion, echinacea, burdock, yellow dock, and licorice. For severe eczema, take one teaspoonful three times a day.

❀ Drink three to four cups daily of red clover tea or my own brand of Petal tea.

Freckles and dark spots

Spots on the skin are generally a form of sun damage and they are difficult to erase. It is important that your doctor checks all spots on the skin regularly for any unusual signs as skin cancer is so prevalent and can be cured if found through regular checks. Minor freckles often worsen when women are taking the contraceptive pill. You may need to find another form of contraception if this is the case.

There are some skin clinics now that have techniques such as peeling masks that can lessen spotty effects on the skin. Make sure you go to a reputable clinic and do not be a guinea pig for any techniques until they are well tried. You can discuss this with your doctor or naturopath.

Foot and nail fungus

This is a very difficult problem to treat naturally. Any fungus likes to live on yeasty foods and sugar so these must be eliminated from the diet.

Treatment

- Use a capsule of acidophilus three times a day before meals to adjust the natural flora in your digestive tract.

- A garlic tablet three times a day helps to kill fungus.

- Use tea-tree oil in cream or liquid form twice daily. Apply externally. If it stings dilute the liquid. One drop of tea-tree oil consumed with half a glass of water has been used by some clients with success. Use one drop once a day and continue no longer than six weeks.

- Sometimes, if the affected area bleeds, an antibiotic must be used, but make sure you follow the treatments recommended above and address any underlying problems.

Fabulous feet

Use a buffer daily under the shower to remove dead skin from the soles. For dry feet, take evening primrose oil or include half an avocado in your diet daily. Take vitamin E, 300 IU daily. If your feet are dry (but not itchy), use a rich foot cream such as sorbolene or lanolin, obtainable from any pharmacist. If they are cracked and itchy, you may have a fungal infection. Wipe the area with tea-tree oil products, which are wonderful for getting rid of fungus, but you must be committed to doing this daily for three to four months.

Psoriasis

This condition is often inherited and can flare up under stress and during seasons when airborne allergens increase histamine levels. Psoriasis will also flare up when your immune system is run down by work overload, travelling, or sleep deprivation. Preventative measures can be taken to decrease the reaction.

Help take the pressure off your immune system by coming off yeast products four weeks *before* spring. Eliminate cheeses, yeasty breads, wine, vinegar, and refined sugars. In these four weeks, take one garlic tablet, two evening primrose oil capsules, one echinacea tablet, and one vitamin C tablet with bioflavonoids (500 mg of each) after each meal. Heavy partying and overloading the liver with alcohol, rich food and recreational drugs can also aggravate the problem. You may consider doing a liver and immune system detox from time to time to clean out any toxins. To keep the liver working at its optimum function, it is advisable to stay on the vital living program (see chapter 11).

Treatment

Follow the practices for dry skin (pages 11–12) and incorporate these supplements.

- Three capsules of omega–3 and –6 oils three times a day until the psoriasis is improved and then cut back to two capsules three times a day.

❀ One vitamin E capsule 500 IU daily. If you have high
blood pressure, check with your doctor with regard to
the dose.

❀ Two bioflavonoid tablets three times a day. These tablets
are made from rutin and hesperidin, which are natural
anti-inflammatory substances.

❀ One complex vitamin B tablet once a day.

❀ Psoriasis is an immune deficiency problem, so boost the
system by taking a combined tablet of echinacea and
andrographis (see page 63). Take two tablets once a day
for at least three months.

❀ Apply a cream made from a base of sorbolene and
vitamin E.

❀ Do not include yeast in your diet until the skin is
70 percent improved and then introduce yeast only
every fourth day.

Hair care

For healthy hair it's important to use a high quality shampoo and a weekly protein pack on the hair. Try to minimize heavy colorings on your hair and discuss alternatives with your hairdresser, such as more natural products that don't include heavy bleaches and chemicals. Stress also plays a major part in how your hair looks. Try to eat regular meals or include nourishing snacks such as shakes or protein soups, as well as some chicken, fish, or legume paste in your diet.

A high protein intake is essential to remedy brittle and breaking hair follicles. For women whose hair is dull and dry, I often prescribe a protein drink made from a tablespoon of soya, rice, or whole milk protein, mixed with water or milk of your choice. Add one teaspoonful of acidophilus powder to assist digestion, which facilitates absorption and metabolism of nutrients. Take this daily. I also recommend the following supplements for natural hair care.

❦ One mineral tablet with calcium, magnesium, and zinc (50–100 mg of each) and one complex vitamin B per day is good for strengthening hair.

❀ Silica is a mineral that is vital for good hair and nails. Chew two small tablets, two to three times a day. Buy the homeopathic forms available from health stores.

❀ If you are breastfeeding and your hair is brittle and your milk supply low, try taking alfalfa tablets, one after each meal, as this herb is high in trace minerals and helps milk supply and hair.

Alopecia

Total or partial hair loss (known as alopecia) can often happen after the birth of a child or even during pregnancy. Trauma, stress, and menopause can also aggravate alopecia. I have seen cases of hair loss after car accidents, divorce, and the loss of a loved one. Sometimes severe cases are inherited. It is important to boost your immune system at this time (follow the treatment for psoriasis on pages 20–21), and to see a naturopath for individual assessment.

Nail care

Nails are a telltale sign of a woman's health and grooming. I often advise my patients to have a regular manicure or to set aside time each week to apply a nutrition cream to keep nails strong and shiny. Here are some other simple suggestions to care for your nails.

- Follow the nutrition program outlined for skin and hair.

- Carry a handcream in your bag and use it frequently to moisturize.

- Make sure you use gloves when using cleaning fluids or gardening.

- For very dry nail beds, apply lanolin cream at night. This is good for those with eczema under or around the nail bed.

- For fungus under the nail bed, apply a weak solution of tea-tree oil with cotton wool each night. Eliminate all yeasty foods from your diet so the fungus is starved of food. If there is bleeding under the nail bed, check with your doctor as the infection may be bacterial.

These supplements can successfully improve nail quality:

- One calcium, magnesium, and zinc mineral tablet after each meal until improvement.
- One acidophilus capsule before each meal to assist the digestion of protein and minerals.
- One vitamin B supplement if you are stressed or anxious and a nail-biter.

White marks on nails

This can be a sign of a number of health issues but generally indicates that the body is not absorbing minerals correctly (calcium, magnesium, zinc, and trace minerals). I often find this with women who have poor digestion and absorption in the stomach and bowel.

Treatment

❧ You must address any digestion issues (see pages 37–41).

❧ Supplement with one mineral tablet (see page 25) twice a day.

❧ If you have constipation take a fiber powder such as Metamucil daily, but don't use this for extended periods.

❧ Check your iron levels as this will assist in your overall metabolism and your absorption of minerals.

❧ Include some dairy products if you are not allergic to them. I suggest low-fat cheese and yogurt or you can try goat's yogurt and cheese.

❧ Eating six almonds daily can also give you some more trace minerals.

2

Your ideal weight

WOMEN COME in all shapes and sizes and most women are happiest when they find their correct weight within the spectrum. Always remember that it is not simply a matter of absolute weight, but of proportion and of your inherited bone and body structure. Some women are naturally lighter and slimmer than others. For example, French women are inherently smaller than Fijian women. However, all women look attractive and sexy if their bodies are in proportion to their structures.

Whatever you do, don't crash diet. It will only bring long-term disappointment. Instead, start by throwing out all the junk food in your cupboards, including cordials, sugary snacks, diet and carbonated drinks, chocolates, sweets, and white flour products; and hide the alcohol. Make sure you have a blood test to check your sugar levels, and for diabetes or thyroid problems. If all of these are clear, your lifestyle and habits must be assessed. Poor bowel habits, long-term stress, hormonal imbalance, and a history of fad dieting can all be major players when it comes to weight gain.

If you are trying to lose weight or to maintain your ideal weight, there are two critical factors:

- you must not use quick fixes and/or extreme dieting;
- you must be consistent in sticking to a healthy eating program and consuming 20 percent less food than normal.

The most successful path to weight loss is to replace those not so healthy foods in your diet with recommended foods (see the vital living program, chapter 11); for example, where you would normally include bread in a meal, replace it with rice and vegetables. You should also include plenty of healthy, low-fat snacks in your day. That way you'll never be starving and won't need to binge on junk food.

Weight problems in many women are caused not only by an overindulgence in fatty foods but also by an insulin imbalance. Many women eat far too much refined sugar: chocolates, cookies, soft drinks, and alcohol. All these foods put an overload on the pancreas, which has to release insulin to metabolize sugars.

Eating a diet high in sugars and carbohydrates means a critical imbalance occurs, where the body stores sugars rather than burning them up. In order to accomplish the desired weight reduction, you must cut right back on breads, pastas, cookies, cakes, and refined sugars (carbonated drinks and chocolate, and sugar in tea and coffee). When eliminating these foods from your diet, a detox is vital. (You may wish to refer to my previous book, *Detox*, which has step-by-step guidelines for three-day detoxes. Then follow the maintenance diet for six weeks. You will be surprised how well it will work for you without extreme dieting.)

Steps to weight loss

Problems with the bowel can be one reason for a bloated stomach and sluggish metabolism, both of which exacerbate weight problems. In an initial step to stabilize or lower your weight, concentrate on maintaining a healthy bowel.

🌸 For healthy bowel flora and regular bowel movements, include a teaspoon of psyllium husks on your cereal in the morning and cut out refined white breads and heavy starches such as white rice and potatoes. Avoid pastries and puddings. Yellow cheese such as cheddar can cause constipation, so should be avoided by women who do not have regular bowel motions.

❀ Include wholemeal fibers on a daily basis: brown rice, grainy wholemeal breads, and high-fiber cereal. Also include raw foods such as carrots, lettuce, cucumbers, beetroot, and celery.

❀ Take a yogurt daily that contains acidophilus (a natural flora), which is essential for balancing the regular bacteria in the bowel and therefore assisting digestion.

❀ For those craving sugar, a small snack of natural crackers or rye biscuits, or fruit can be eaten between meals. These snacks are not calorie-loaded, but they are satisfying and stop the temptation to eat junk food. One to two pieces of fruit are good, but sometimes fruit increases appetite. A yogurt with the fruit will slow down the sugar digestion and maintain energy levels for two to three hours.

❧ When tempted to reach for sugary snacks, cakes, and refined food with hidden fats (butter, chocolate, salami, and fried foods), try one of the following: a snack such as soup, a protein drink, a thin slice of bread or a wholemeal biscuit with some low-fat white cheese or a slice of chicken or ham or a legume paste with no added fat.

❧ Exercise three to four times a week to keep the metabolism burning unwanted fat and wastes.

❧ Maintain a high fluid intake of filtered water, herbal tea (three to four glasses of each per day), and fresh raw juices (one vegetable and one fruit juice daily).

❧ Eat very small meals frequently to help with weight control. Liquid foods such as soup and raw juices also help. Gently steamed vegetables can be eaten anytime, as they never add fat or excess fluid.

❧ You may wish to buy a soya protein powder or a rice-based protein powder to use as a quick pick-up drink if you are busy with children or at work. Use a heaped teaspoonful in a glass of water or low-fat milk. Include a fruit in this drink for flavor and health.

❧ If you have reflux (which is too high an acid content in the stomach), a hiatus hernia or some inflammation of the oesophagus, then two capsules of slippery elm powder before each meal work wonders.

Supplementation

For anyone who's overweight, I recommend the following supplements.

❧ Acidophilus capsules: one to two before each meal to assist digestion and a bloated stomach.

❧ B_6 tablet (100 mg): one after each meal to assist metabolism, moods, and fluid retention.

❧ A magnesium powder or tablet with chromium (which controls cravings for sugar). Take a teaspoonful two to three times a day or one tablet after each meal.

See your health store for the best dosage to combat your sugar cravings.

🐾 Iron and B$_{12}$ supplement: one each per day. If a blood test shows your iron levels are very low, then your doctor or naturopath will prescribe a higher dose. There is a liquid iron supplement available—the dose is two teaspoonfuls twice a day.

🐾 A complex mineral tablet containing calcium, magnesium, zinc and potassium. Take one tablet morning and evening. This is particularly important for adolescent girls between the ages of 12 and 18 as it is during this time that their bones develop to full strength.

🐾 Use a mild herbal laxative (senna or Metamucil) if constipated. Take one teaspoonful once or twice a day.

🐾 To control sugar cravings, make a tonic from equal amounts of dandelion root (to clean the liver), bilberry (to normalize blood sugar), St Mary's thistle (to help fat metabolism in the liver), and dandelion leaves (to reduce fluid retention). Take a teaspoonful three times a day in a glass of water for at least two to three months or until your eating habits have improved and your weight has stabilized.

❧ If you have no heart disease, chew pure hard licorice to help sugar cravings. Licorice tea, such as my Triple E tea, can also be drunk freely between meals to take away the desire to eat sweet things, especially in the afternoon.

Exercise

It is difficult for busy women to include regular exercise in their lives, but it is essential to assist with weight loss and more generally with a sense of well being. You may speed up your diet program by power walking for an hour three times a week. Two to three times a week also include some form of aerobic exercise to increase the heart rate. Try aerobic classes, swimming, bike riding, jazz ballet classes, or anything that makes you sweat for an hour.

Cellulite

This type of fat is a chronic problem for women.
It seems to be connected to hormonal imbalance
and inadequate exercise. There is no wonder cream or
drug that will fix cellulite. In my experience, the best
way of discouraging more cellulite (and reducing what
you already have) is to increase water intake or herbal
tea intake to at least eight glasses a day. Make sure
you exercise three to four times a week. Really do it
and don't just think about it. During your "thinking"
time the cellulite is also thinking about getting worse!

Hunger repressants

Do not use hunger repressants as they cause damage
to the natural digestive enzymes that are vital in
breaking down proteins, fats, and sugars. If you have
poor digestion an enzyme tablet, available from health
stores, can be taken with your meal.

Gluten-free eating

If you are a very disciplined person, a fast and healthy way to lose weight is to remove gluten from your diet completely. Gluten is a sticky substance found in all grains except rice, so this means you must eliminate all breads, pastas, cookies, croissants, cakes, and even couscous and buckwheat. Sometimes soya products contain gluten. Do this for the time it takes you to achieve your optimum weight (the weight at which you feel comfortable and healthy). I find that following a gluten-free diet for six to eight weeks has a remarkable effect on weight loss.

You may wish to use gluten-free bread or pasta but they are generally not that appealing and you will have better weight-loss results if you include vegetables, rice, and one or two potatoes instead for your carbohydrate balance with your choice of protein.

Extreme bloating and bowel irregularities may indicate gluten intolerance. You may either see a doctor to refer you for further tests, or stop all gluten products. It is a very difficult program to follow but well worth the three-month trial to see how much better you feel and how flat your stomach becomes.

Sugar cravings

The herb gymnema (*Gymnema sylvestre*) grows in India, Sri Lanka, China, Japan, Malaysia, Indonesia, and Vietnam. Its Hindi name means "sugar destroyer" as it has the amazing property of suppressing cravings for sugar. It is wonderful for those suffering from diabetes and sugar cravings. Ideally, it should be used throughout the day, every two to three hours. With a dropper, place 1–2 ml of the liquid extract on the tongue. Leave for one minute then rinse off with water.

Bloating

Almost every woman I see as a client complains of bloating. This may not be the major reason for their visit but it always comes up in conversation. Through my personal experiences in treating women I have found that bloating is possibly one of the most distressing and frustrating conditions as most women do not know how to address it.

Generally the two main causes of bloating are:

- an overload of yeast and fermented foods in the diet; and
- hormonal imbalance, particularly seven to ten days before the period.

You will have a much flatter stomach if you follow the procedures below faithfully. These have had excellent results for women of all age groups. If you have the discipline and the desire to obtain this goal then it is possible, and I have seen wonderful results in many of my clients. But the rewards do not come lightly. You must set aside six to twelve months for long and lasting results.

Treatment

❧ Eliminate all yeasty foods, including bread, pasta, cheese, cakes, and cookies; also refined desserts, sweets such as chocolate, white sugars, rich sauces, and wine. (I allow my clients two slices of yeast-free bread daily.)

❧ Over a three-month period eat only fresh vegetables, fresh fruits, and a variety of protein. Continue for

another three months for better results. If you are
desperate for pasta or a sugary dessert, indulge once a
week but take two acidophilus tablets afterwards to
eliminate the yeast and to balance the natural flora of
your digestive tract.

❧ Drink at least eight glasses of pure fresh water daily and
include organic herbal teas and one or two raw juices
daily away from food.

❧ After the initial three-month period, include rice at least
every second day for your carbohydrate balance. (Thai
food is a good example of combining rice with protein
and vegetables.)

❧ For your ongoing regime, use wholemeal grains and
cereals for breakfast with skim or soya milk. If you suffer
constipation, wholemeal foods will help to regulate your
bowel naturally. If you need extra help, add a teaspoonful
of psyllium husks to food once or twice a day or see your
naturopath.

❧ Take a low-fat yogurt in the morning and at night or two acidophilus capsules before each meal.

❧ Take two evening primrose oil capsules morning and night to assist bowel motions and hormonal balance (see also chapter 6).

❧ Stop any vitamin or herb that is aggravating your digestion.

❧ Move your bowel once a day. If this is not happening, take an extra two acidophilus capsules before bed. If still sluggish, include senna capsules that you can obtain from a health store. Take one or two after dinner.

❧ Do 20 to 40 stomach crunches daily to tone stomach muscles. Lie on your back with your knees bent, feet on the floor. Then gently use your stomach muscles to raise your torso towards your knees. Begin slowly and build on these exercises. They also tighten the bladder muscles for women.

Cutting out carbohydrates altogether can be difficult, even if it is only for a short time. Try cutting back on them slowly and use the vital living program (chapter 11) as a guide. This will certainly be a step in the right direction. Your results may be a little slower if you do occasionally include bread or sugar or the odd glass of wine, but you will certainly become aware of how your stomach reacts to these products.

Wheat grass juice

This juice is extraordinary. It contains 90 minerals out of the 102 possible trace minerals found in rich soil. It is about 20 percent protein and has trace amounts of B_{12} (excellent for vegetarians and those who lack energy). It contains many digestive enzymes, which are vital to cell function and assist the body to detox from drugs, cancer, Hepatitis B, chronic fatigue, metal poisoning, joint problems, and all digestive problems. It is best mixed with water or carrot juice as it can make you feel a little nauseated in the beginning due to its powerful antioxidant properties. It is worth it. Persevere. Incorporate a teaspoonful of it, fresh or powdered, daily.

Food intolerance

If you are extremely bloated and suffer constipation and/or diarrhea and unpleasant flatulence, you may be allergic to certain foods (see also pages 67–70). Keep a food diary for six weeks by recording each meal you have. Note which foods cause you to bloat. Cut these foods out of your diet for the next six weeks and then introduce them one at a time. If you notice that you are aggravated badly after a certain food, you will know to stop it for at least another three months. Try the food again in small amounts, as often as you can tolerate it.

Anorexia and bulimia

These eating disorders occur particularly in young women and are difficult to treat by naturopathic methods alone. The condition is psychological, rooted in emotional trauma, peer-group pressure, drug abuse, and body image. I recommend working with your doctor, psychologist, and naturopath.

For anyone who suffers from this condition, whey powder makes an excellent protein drink that's gentle on the stomach. It's not a heavy, fattening drink.

3

Depression, anxiety, insomnia

STRESS, TRAUMA, hormonal imbalance, drug abuse, and the pressures of family and work life can all bring about the very real and disturbing symptoms of depression, anxiety, and insomnia. These three conditions often go hand in hand and in the twenty-first century they are a widespread problem that affects females, young and old.

Make a diary of your moods and see if your mood changes when you eat poorly or around the time of your period. If you're only getting these symptoms seven to ten days prior to your period, they could indicate pre-menstrual tension (see chapter 6). If your symptoms are related to menopause, then refer to chapter 7.

Preventative program

Sugars leach out important minerals that are essential for the well being of our nerves. One way of keeping depression and anxiety at bay is to avoid the rapid highs and lows following excess sugar intake. Remove all the foods that tend to cause sugar level disturbances such as sweets, candies, chocolates, cakes, cookies, and alcohol, and fried foods that overload the liver's detoxification pathways. Allergies can often bring on or aggravate mood swings and anxiety attacks, so if you become aware that certain foods cause this reaction, note this in your diary and eliminate them too.

You will be surprised how you can start to take control of some of your life through these simple measures.

Follow the vital living program (see chapter 11) and concentrate on the following:

- Eat five small meals a day with plenty of rice; fresh and raw vegetables; fruits; quality proteins such as fish, chicken, eggs, tofu, and legumes; and red meat three times a week.
- Eat grainy breads with a protein snack on top to boost

your energy. Use yogurt and low-fat milk to boost calcium levels, which will settle the nerves.

- Drink chamomile, Petal, or vervain tea throughout the day as well as water and fresh juices. These teas are traditionally proven to relax and soothe.
- Take a mineral tablet with calcium and magnesium twice a day.
- Take one complex vitamin B per day to assist stress and moods. If you are very anxious, try taking one at lunch, too.
- Take one St John's wort tablet per day to assist low-level anxiety attacks and stress. If you are staying awake at night worrying, take one to two passionflower or valerian tablets before bed, with a glass of skim milk to help digest them.

Exercise

Exercise is vital in the treatment of all forms of depression and anxiety. Research has shown that some form of aerobic exercise for 30 minutes a day (this includes fast walking) increases the production of a vital chemical called phenylethylamine, which is similar in structure to amphetamines (the substances found in antidepressant medication). This natural chemical is sometimes used clinically to treat depression.

In fact, in a study at Indiana University, a review of all clinical evidence concluded that a 20-minute brisk walk (at a pace that left the subjects breathing hard but not exhausted) was the best way to boost mental health. The psychological benefits they discovered were comparable to the sort of improvements expected from a course of psychotherapy.

Some scientists believe that in the long-term, regular jogging or gym sessions could lead to the regeneration of adult brain cells, which has always been thought an impossibility.

Depression

Talk to your naturopath or local doctor to obtain a proper diagnosis. If you decide to take natural medicine, the following program is advisable:

❧ L-tyrosine (an amino acid): one tablet after each meal.

❧ St John's wort tablets: one after breakfast and one after dinner.

❧ Magnesium tablets or powder: 200–300 mg three times a day (relaxant for the nerves and muscles).

❧ Calcium: one 500–1000 mg tablet three times a day (excellent for nerves and depression).

❧ Vitamin B complex (50–100 mg of each B): one after each meal. Do not take within four hours of sleep as it can keep you awake.

When you are feeling better, cut the doses by half and stay on them until you feel confident in your lifestyle and happiness.

If you are very severely depressed because of trauma, a great loss in your life, or even drug abuse, there are excellent antidepressants now available that are non-addictive. They can be taken for the short-term until you are over the critical phase of your problem. You must not take St John's wort if you are on a medically prescribed antidepressant.

The feel-good factor

Serotonin is the most important of the "feel good" hormones in the brain (Prozac and other antidepressants work on increasing levels of serotonin), and there are ways of increasing this vital "feel good" hormone naturally.

Herbs that help the body increase serotonin and therefore cope with stress are:

- St John's wort
- Siberian ginseng and panax ginseng
- Gotu kola
- Shisandra

Make a tonic of equal parts of these herbs and take a teaspoonful two to three times a day for at least three to six months.

Low melatonin levels are also associated with depression. This natural hormone is produced in deep sleep and has now been shown to have healing effects, possibly because when the body is allowed to sleep deeply, the repair of tissues and immune system can take place correctly. Adequate sleep or melatonin supplements can improve your life dramatically.

I recommend that you try the preventative program and the vitamin supplements together with St John's wort before you resort to medical antidepressants. Yoga, meditation, and finding the right job are also very important in feeling good about yourself. If you are having problems with your family life, work through the issues with a friend or counselor. There is help available.

Anxiety

Many people suffer anxiety in our hectic world. It can manifest itself as mild anxiety or as panic attacks and overwhelming nervousness. Anxiety can be a symptom of PMT, experienced two weeks to ten days before the menstrual cycle begins (see chapter 6). You can actually take control of your anxiety, and here are some suggestions for preventing it.

❦ Diet plays an important role. Eat regular meals, which will keep your blood sugar levels consistent therefore preventing mood swings. See the vital living program (chapter 11) and use the ideas for healthy snacks to also avoid hypoglycemia (low blood sugar level).

✿ Those who don't eat many dairy products must take calcium and magnesium supplements or begin to eat more yogurt, low-fat milk and/or cheese, and include almonds and sesame seeds in their daily diet.

✿ Avoid heavily spiced foods.

✿ Eliminate caffeine from your diet. This is found in coffee, tea, cola drinks, and chocolate.

✿ Stop all recreational drugs and cigarette smoking.

✿ During stressful times, watch your breathing. Notice when it becomes quite shallow. Take five to ten deep breaths. This allows more oxygen into the lungs and relaxes the mind.

✿ A homeopathic remedy called Rescue Remedy (see page 53) is helpful for shock or mild panic attacks during stressful moments. Take five drops every five minutes until you feel better.

Treatment

Each of these treatments can be used individually. Try them one at a time to find the one most suitable for you.

🌺 Follow the treatment for depression (see pages 46–48), but use only a low-dose vitamin B as this can sometimes aggravate anxiety.

🌺 Drink my Petal or vervain tea three times a day. They are wonderful for calming the nerves.

🌺 Take one passionflower tablet after each meal. This herb is excellent for anxiety.

🌺 Valerian tablets can also be tried for anxiety. Take half to one tablet after each meal. If it makes you too sleepy, use passionflower instead.

🌺 Follow the vital living program in chapter 11.

🌺 If you do not like tablets, a tonic made from the following herbs is excellent for anxiety: equal parts of

vervain, passionflower, chamomile, and St John's wort.
Take one teaspoonful two to three times a day in half a
glass of water.

Panic attacks

We do not know why these occur as they are not all related to
stress and anxiety.

Some of my clients say they only experienced them after the
birth of their children, which could point to hormonal
imbalance. Other women report experiencing them after a virus,
especially if they suffer chronic fatigue. Panic attacks can come at
any time. There is often a feeling of overwhelming dread just
beforehand. The heartbeat is elevated and the individual can
experience severe sweating.

According to the individual and their circumstances treatment varies widely. Worry and anxiety about daily living can be an
underlying cause and it is important that issues worrying you are
addressed. Eliminate as many stressors as possible, and organize
your life to give you greater self-esteem and happiness.

Treatment

Natural remedies also have a place in the treatment of panic attacks and it is often wise to try them before resorting to stronger medication.

- ❧ Magnesium, a muscle relaxant, is vital regardless of the cause: take a chelated tablet of 100 mg, three times a day. Doses can be larger, but a naturopath should advise.

- ❧ St John's wort: one or two tablets a day. Check with your doctor if you are on other medication.

- ❧ Rescue Remedy, a homeopathic medicine made from the essence of flowers: take five drops under the tongue every five minutes during an attack.

- ❧ Calcium is essential for nerves and should be supplemented, especially if you are not ingesting calcium foods in your diet. Begin with 500 mg a day and increase the dosage according to your doctor or naturopath.

- ❧ Evening primrose oil is useful in some cases: 3000 mg a day.

❀ Slow breathing exercises during an attack can be miraculous. Take ten deep breaths to slow down the heart rate.

❀ Regular yoga classes can assist.

❀ Pursue new hobbies, contact old friends, and instigate a change of job or even a change of environment such as moving house. A great holiday is always a key to help accumulated stress.

Insomnia

Sleeping patterns depend very much on your psychological state but there are natural ways to ensure you have a good night's sleep. It's simply a question of making subtle shifts in your daily routine and being aware of what may be causing the problem. Stress, worry, anxiety, jet lag, and illness can all cause insomnia. Going to bed on a full stomach or soon after a large meal can also contribute to a restless night. Insomnia can often exacerbate itself because the more you worry about not sleeping, the more you'll be kept awake worrying.

Treatment

❧ Don't have any caffeine (coffee, tea, chocolate) at least eight to ten hours before sleeping.

❧ Avoid having a heavy meal before bed. Eat only freshly cooked vegetables with fish or a light white meat protein. Red meat, rich sauces, and alcohol will stimulate digestion and the mind. If you are eating these foods, have them at least four to five hours before you go to bed.

❧ Try a calcium tablet (500 mg) before going to bed. Often this will change your sleeping habits by relaxing the nerves. A magnesium tablet (300 mg) can be tried if the calcium is not helping.

❧ Have a cup of organic chamomile tea half an hour before bed to relax the brain.

❧ For persistent insomnia, try Mexican valerian tablets. Take one to two tablets with a glass of warm skim milk or chamomile tea 20 minutes before retiring.

❧ Melatonin tablets (3 mg) assist many people and must only be taken before bedtime (one tablet daily).

❧ If anxiety and worry are keeping you awake, you may wish to follow the advice in the anxiety program (see pages 51–52) until you are better.

❧ Twenty minutes of quiet time and meditation before bed can be very helpful for those with high stress.

4

Boosting the immune system

WHETHER YOU SUFFER mildly or severely from a depleted immune system, it is absolutely essential that you boost your immunity before the onslaught of winter or travel to a colder climate. If you have suffered from major bronchial and asthmatic problems it may take two winters for your system to strengthen, but rest assured that preventative measures do work. For the cost of a few simple daily routines, your quality of life can be so much greater.

Signs that your natural immunity is low are regular colds and flus, bronchitis, allergies, asthma, sinus problems, dermatitis (skin irritations), and cystitis.

Preventative program

Begin this program at least six to eight weeks before winter sets in. If you are a chronic sufferer of low immunity, then the following routines should be included in your diet for six months of the year.

- Drink a glass of warm water with freshly squeezed lemon juice, with honey if desired, every morning.

- Drink a freshly squeezed orange juice daily.

- Stay away from mucus-forming foods, such as milk and cheese, and large quantities of bread (use rice instead), carbonated drinks, chocolate, and cakes.

- Eat as many fresh vegetables and fruits as you can daily, and include fish high in omega oils (tinned salmon, tuna, or sardines) three times a week. They are good for preventing chest complaints.

- Eat plenty of thick homemade soups with fresh vegetables, barley and split peas.

❀ Use garlic and onions as frequently as possible, and include horseradish when you can.

❀ Include spices in your food, especially ginger and cayenne.

❀ Drink peppermint, fresh mint, or ginger tea daily.

❀ Keep alcohol to a minimum, especially champagne and white wines, which are high in additives. These can trigger asthma attacks.

❀ Make sure your iron levels are not low. Ask your doctor for a check well before winter.

Preventative supplements

❀ Combination garlic and horseradish: one tablet after each meal.

❀ Vitamin C with bioflavonoids (500 mg of each): one tablet, twice daily.

❧ An immune-boosting tablet made from either echinacea, cats claw, astragalus and andrographis or any combination. Ask your health store for this supplement. These herbs work in combination to maintain a healthy immune system and fight viral and bacterial infections. Take one tablet, twice a day.

**A s t r a g a l u s
(*A s t r a g a l u s   m e m b r a n a c e u s*)**
This is an official herb in Chinese and Japanese pharmacopoeias and grows well in the mountainous districts of Iran and Iraq. In Chinese medicine astragalus is well respected as a tonic to assist *qi* (energy) and blood (nutrition). In the western world it is used for treating long-term chronic infections. It boosts the immune system after chemotherapy, radiotherapy, and surgery.

The common cold or flu

Follow the preventative measures described on pages 58–59 while you are suffering from a cold or flu and continue for at least a month after the illness has passed. When you're under the weather, follow these instructions for a speedy recovery.

🌿 Make a drink of hot water, lemon juice, honey, and freshly grated ginger (one teaspoonful) and drink at least four to five times a day while you are in the severe stages of the flu, and two to three times a day for a week later.

🌿 Keep fluids high using the drink just described and hot peppermint tea. My Summer Delight tea and the flu tea (see page 62) are ideal.

🌿 Your appetite will be reduced so drink chicken and vegetable broths and eat fresh salads with a light protein such as fish or tofu.

🌿 Use inhalations of peppermint and eucalyptus oils or simply rub some old-fashioned Vicks Vapo-Rub into the chest area regularly.

🌿 Stay in bed and rest for at least 24 to 48 hours. You may sweat, which is a good sign.

An amazing flu tea

This is a traditionally proven tea for colds, flu, and fevers. It's safe for everyone over five years. Make up a batch of the following dried herbs, obtainable from health stores:

- 2 tablespoons yarrow
- 2 tablespoons peppermint
- 2 tablespoons eyebright
- 1 teaspoon ginger
- 1 teaspoon cinnamon
- ½ to 1 teaspoon cayenne powder

Combine herbs, then add one teaspoonful of mixture to a cup of boiling water. Drink hot with honey as often as possible.

Supplements for the common cold

Vitamin C with bioflavonoids (500 mg each): one every three to four hours.

Garlic tablet or fresh garlic (one clove): one every three to four hours.

An immune-stimulant herbal formula either in tablet or liquid form that includes echinacea, cats claw, licorice, ginger, peppermint, and andrographis (a herbalist can make this for you). If using as a liquid, add a teaspoonful to half a glass of warm water every three to four hours. Use equal parts of each herb but only a quarter of the amount of ginger, as its taste will overwhelm. Or take a tablet every three hours until better, then three times a day for two to three weeks to boost your immune system.

Andrographis (*Andrographis paniculata*)

Traditionally know as the "king of bitters" in India where it is highly valued as a medicine, this herb is classed as a cold remedy and therefore used to clear heat from the body especially in the lungs and respiratory organs. It has excellent anti-inflammatory properties and works well in counteracting bacterial and viral infections like the common cold and viral throats and fevers. Andrographis has been found to be very helpful when used long term against stubborn urinary tract infections. Do not use during pregnancy.

Mouth ulcers and cold sores

Mouth ulcers and cold sores are a classic sign that you are generally run down. They can also indicate that your system is too acidic. Stop all citrus fruits, tomatoes, wines, white sugar, spices, and carbonated drinks. Build your immune system by taking one tablet of echinacea daily for three to four months. Also include a multivitamin with added minerals and an antioxidant tablet. For immediate treatment of ulcers, combine 2 ml each of myrrh and sage with warm water. Gargle and spit it out. Repeat three times a day. For cold sores, buy some liquid extract of *Melissa officinalis* and dab on the affected area three to four times a day. It works quickly to dry it up.

Asthma

The preventative program on pages 58–59 is essential in the long term for asthma sufferers. Asthma can be caused by many different triggers. Some sufferers are allergy prone (see chapter 5), some are subject to a general weakness of the immune system and some are both. A naturopath and herbalist can often get to the source of the problem and can suggest natural vitamins and herbs that can be taken alongside any prescription medicine from your doctor. Remember it is always wise to let your doctor know what supplements you are taking.

If you suffer from asthma, follow these simple and safe recommendations to boost your immune system.

🌿 Follow the acute treatment program for flu and colds (see page 61), as this program is safe with drugs such as Ventolin.

🌿 As a preventative tonic, use a tablet or liquid made from boswellia, andrographis, licorice, thyme, and peppermint—three times a day. These herbs are marvellous to help open the bronchial pathways.

🦋 Swimming is a wonderful preventative measure for asthmatics and has shown good results.

Asthma has increased in recent years and is becoming more severe in children. It is one of the ten most common reasons for seeing a general practitioner. About 30 percent of all Americans will have respiratory symptoms consistent with asthma at some time in their lives.

Cats claw
(*Uncaria tomentosa*)

This is one of the most celebrated plants of the Ashaninka Indians, the indigenous people of the Peruvian central rainforest. Cats claw became a threatened species in 1994 due to its popularity as an immune-enhancing herb, especially for HIV infections, carcinoma and auto-immune disorders. Now, it is protected by special legislation in Peru. We use the stem bark as it is illegal to harvest or disturb the root. Cats claw is wonderful for post-viral conditions such as chronic fatigue and long-term flu and viral infections. I find it works very well with echinacea, astragalus, and boswellia.

5

Allergies and intolerances

IN OUR HIGHLY chemical world, we can react to foods, to dust, to household cleaners—even fragrances. It's important to identify what's irritating you and to avoid it if possible.

Food

After eating certain foods, you may experience an upset or bloated stomach (see page 37), diarrhea, skin rashes or itchiness, tiredness, irritability, anxiety, moodiness, or constipation. If symptoms are constantly severe after the same foods, you may have a food allergy. If they are mild and don't happen all the time, it could be a food intolerance. A blood test from your doctor or specialized allergy clinic will help diagnose any allergies. To recover from a food allergy you have little choice but to stay away from the food in question. With a food intolerance, you should be able to eat small amounts of the offending food every three to four days without suffering a reaction.

Treatment for food allergies

❦ If you have a specific food allergy, it's a good idea to complete a short, gentle detox program. For two to three days, eat only a bowl of vegetable soup every two to three hours. In between drink fresh, raw vegetable and fruit juices. If you're hungry, snack on raw vegetables. Get plenty of rest and avoid strenuous exercise. Cut out all vitamins during the detox. After the detox, incorporate the vital living program (see chapter 11) into your life.

❦ Include vitamin C tablets with bioflavonoids (1000 mg), two to three times a day, and take one to two antioxidant tablets per day.

❧ If, by mistake, you eat a food to which you are allergic, follow the vital living program and include the necessary vitamins (see page 68) to get you back on a healthier path.

Treatment for food intolerances

Food intolerances are subtle and it is often difficult to avoid all suspect foods, particularly if you are a highly allergic person. Before you begin this treatment, you should undergo a three-day detox specifically for allergies. This detox will take the overload off the liver, repair the bowel wall, and replace digestive enzymes internally through raw juices, fresh vegetables and by introducing yogurt regularly. Once you have completed the detox, take the following supplements:

❧ One acidophilus capsule before each meal to assist digestion.

❧ A bitter drink such as Campari and soda or the juice of half a lemon in water with a sprig of fresh mint before a meal to help the digestive enzymes.

❧ Two evening primrose oil capsules after each meal or a
teaspoonful of a cold-pressed oil such as safflower,
sunflower, or linseed twice a day if you are having
irregular bowel motions.

Airborne allergies

Seasonal changes can have a profound affect on how you feel.
Pollens are a real problem and they quickly cause a histaminic
reaction. Pollens irritate the lining of the nose and sinuses. The
body compensates by producing phlegm or mucus to offset this
inflammatory process. Symptoms include sneezing, sinus
problems, earaches, coughs, and bronchial conditions and
infections, dizziness, skin rashes, flaky scalp, dry fingernail beds,
red and puffy eyes, and general lethargy.

During high-allergy seasons, keep wine to a minimum as this
will often aggravate symptoms. Three weeks before the seasonal
changes, build up the immune system by taking the following
preventative supplements:

❧ Vitamin C with bioflavonoids (500 mg of each): one combination tablet or a teaspoonful of powder two to three times a day in a glass of water or juice. This strengthens the mucous membranes against airborne foreign bodies in the sinus.

❧ Echinacea tablets: one after each meal to boost immunity.

❧ Garlic, horseradish, and fenugreek: one after each meal. Excellent to 'mop up' excess mucus. The garlic acts as a natural antibacterial agent, helping to keep the sinus and ears clear of infection.

❧ Lots of fresh orange, pineapple, and lemon juice daily: 500 ml of fresh citrus juice per day is ideal during spring.

❧ Ginger and peppermint teas either combined or by themselves: three cups a day. You may add chamomile, which is excellent for allergies, too, and especially relaxing in the evening.

Keep dust from building up around the house and especially sleeping areas. There are special house "dust busters" that you may wish to invest in if you have a family with allergies and asthma. Use eucalyptus cleaning fluids and environmentally friendly household cleaning agents.

Treatment

When you're suffering acutely from airborne allergies, try the following remedies.

- Vitamin C with bioflavonoids (500 mg of each): two tablets or a teaspoonful of the powder in water every three to four hours during the day for the first 48 hours. When you're feeling better, use this dose two to three times a day.

- Euphrasia: one tablet after each meal. This herb is excellent for hay fever and sinus problems.

- Garlic and horseradish tablet (with fenugreek if you can obtain this at your health store): two tablets after each meal until better, then lower the dose to one after each meal.

❧ If you are not allergic to beestings, take a propolis throat spray or lozenges regularly to assist a sore throat.

❧ If you are suffering from a bronchial attack, or a mucous drip that might irritate your bronchials, take a tonic made from equal parts of echinacea, peppermint, elecampane, euphrasia, thyme, wild cherry, and marshmallow: one teaspoonful, three to four times a day in water.

❧ If you have skin rashes, include high doses of evening primrose oil: two to three capsules after each meal.

❧ Place a few drops of peppermint or eucalyptus oil on a cotton handkerchief and breathe it regularly to keep the nasal passageways clear from the pollens in the air.

❧ Ask your local chemist for some soothing eye drops for dry and itchy eyes: use three to four times a day.

Eyebright
(*Euphrasia officinalis*)

An eye bath made from euphrasia is wonderful for sore and irritated eyes from seasonal allergies or other irritation. Make a tea with one teaspoonful of the dried herb and a cup of boiling water in a pot. Let stand for five minutes to draw then strain and pour. Cool and bathe each eye in a fresh bath three times a day. You can drink a cup of the tea two to three times a day too.

6

Hormones

VERY FEW WOMEN are fortunate enough to go through life without some sort of hormonal imbalance. Some women don't even realize that their moods and irritabilities are closely related to their monthly cycles. In order to regulate hormones, you must be aware of how your body feels. Keep a daily diary of moods, weight fluctuations, breast soreness, and anxiety in relation to your cycle. Day one begins on the first day of bleeding and your cycle could be between 28 and 32 days. Some women's cycles follow no particular pattern. Through the diary you can monitor how you are affected physically and mentally at different times.

As hormones are such a huge part of women's health, I have divided this chapter into sections. Once you are aware of the

pattern that your cycles are taking, refer to the individual section
for treatment and ideas to assist you.

Knowing your cycle

Generally a woman ovulates between the tenth and seventeenth
day of her cycle. It is around this time that a woman is most fertile.
To work out the ovulation stage of your particular cycle, deduct
fourteen days from the first day of your last period. For example,
if your cycle is 30 days, then you'll ovulate around day 16 if your
periods are always regular. Often women become pregnant when
they rely on this guidance to calculate their ovulation time but
their periods do not follow a regular pattern. Even a few days
before and after ovulation you must take precautions, as sperm
can live up to 48 hours and sometimes even longer.

Balancing your hormones

❧ Sugar cravings often happen before a period. Eat small
   snacks every few hours or have five to six per day.

❀ Avoid or eliminate sweets containing refined sugar. Eat a piece of fruit instead or a protein snack such as a nut spread on a Rye Vita cracker, a muesli bar, or a handful of almonds with a tub of yogurt.

❀ Make simple carbohydrate snacks for those times when you are really craving heavy starches. Keep some thick barley and vegetable soups in the freezer for quick reheating. Cook a potato and add a filling of avocado or tuna with tomato, basil, and onions.

❀ Yeasty foods such as breads, pasta, and cakes will aggravate a puffy stomach.

❀ Make sure you eat fresh vegetables daily in a range of colors. Raw vegetables are also a great snack. Dipped in a hummus paste they can soothe the cravings of the monthly cycles.

❀ Drink carrot juice with added ginger. Ginger helps relieve period pain. Substitute fresh juices, water, and herbal teas for cordials and carbonated drinks.

❦ Eliminate cigarettes and caffeine and reduce alcohol to a minimum (three to four glasses per week).

❦ White and red wine and champagne contain high levels of sugars and yeast. We often crave these drinks before a period. Substitute with vodka and tonic or Campari and soda, which contain little or no sugar and yeast. Fruit cocktails with an alcohol base are deadly before a period; only use as an occasional special treat.

❦ Exercise, yoga, meditation, and relaxation are vital for a healthy functioning hormonal system.

❦ Stress levels need to be reduced as this has been found to be a factor in infertility. Exercise is a good way of reducing stress, depression, and anxiety (see chapter 3).

Fish oils

Omega-3 oils are what are often referred to as the "fish oils" on labels and in magazines. The omega-3 oils are obtained from cold-water fish—salmon, cod, mackerel, tuna, and sardines—and linseed oil. These unsaturated fatty acids are essential for balancing our good cholesterol HDL and act as an anti-inflammatory for numerous complaints that I refer to throughout this book, especially eczema and PMT. Omega-6 oils are sourced from evening primrose oil and soya oil. They also act as an anti-inflammatory on cell membranes.

It is vital to note here that the omega-3 and -6 oils, or these "good" fats, are an important component of cell membranes and therefore affect the way cells function. Hence in eczema, as well as in arthritis and multiple sclerosis, they act as an anti-inflammatory and help to regenerate cell membrane. They are preventative as well as restorative. When buying these oils in combination it is important that the correct ratio is used. There must be four times more omega-6 than omega-3. Make sure that omega-6 oils are sourced organically and check the farming of the fish oils, through your naturopath or local distributor of the product.

Pre-menstrual tension

PMT is the name for a condition with a variety of symptoms, including irritability, depression, headaches, emotional instability, fluid retention, and breast tenderness, occurring a week to ten days before a period. Some women have complained that these symptoms begin two weeks prior to a period. They find that their lives are severely affected both personally and professionally by these difficult and sometimes uncontrollable symptoms. The liver plays an important role in clearing excess oestrogens in the blood, so decreasing coffee and alcohol and taking a multivitamin B supplement assist in the removal of harmful oestrogens.

Treatment

- Chasteberry: take 50 drops each morning in half a glass of water beginning 14 days prior to your period. Use one tablet each day if you prefer.

- Essential fatty acids in the form of evening primrose oil and fish oil are helpful: one capsule of each three times a day beginning 14 days prior to your period.

- Vitamin E: 250 IU daily.

❀ Magnesium powder: one teaspoonful twice a day or one 200 mg tablet three times a day. Take for 14 days prior to the commencement of your period, especially if you are subject to cramps and headaches. Magnesium is a relaxant for the muscle tissue of the uterus and thus a great help in discomfort. Take a 200 mg tablet every four hours if you have pain or very severe irritability in PMT.

❀ Chamomile or Petal tea: three cups daily, or choose a tea that suits you. Dandelion root tea assists liver function and bowel movements. Ginger tea daily will assist circulation to the uterus, and has been traditionally used to assist in the discomfort and pain associated with PMT.

❀ If you eat very few foods containing calcium and have insomnia before a period, take 500–1000 mg of calcium before bed. This not only soothes the nerves but is a wonderful sleeping aid.

❀ If you experience anxiety, take a tablet of passionflower herb two to three times a day. Check with your health store about the standard dosage.

❦ During the pre-menstrual phase depression can be a significant issue as serotonin levels can drop (see page 48). Take two St John's wort tablets a day to assist in depressive symptoms, combined with exercise and rest (see also chapter 3).

❦ If you're craving sugar, chew on hard licorice root three times a day and follow the points in the vital living program (see chapter 11).

❦ If you have tender or swollen breasts, take vitamin B_6 (300–600 mg daily), which can reduce the swelling enormously before a period.

Period pain

Period pain (dysmenorrhoea) often begins on the first day of the period and stops 24 hours later. Young girls between the ages of 13 and 18 often experience this problem, which frequently disappears after the birth of a first child. In many cases, the pain responds very well to natural medicine. If you have little or no results from this treatment, you can discuss with your doctor the options of pain killers or the contraceptive pill, which can relieve severe symptoms.

Treatment

Follow the treatment for PMT on pages 80–82 and include the following:

🌿 A magnesium tablet of 200 mg every one to two hours for severe pain.

🌿 Ginger tea every hour.

🌿 A tonic (one teaspoonful four times a day or every four hours) made from equal parts of cramp bark, blue cohosh, black cohosh, dong quai, and peppermint. Ginger should be added if you are not taking ginger tea. Add 10 percent ginger to the tonic as this herb is very strong and spicy when taken in concentrated amounts. This tonic can be taken three times a day for a week before your period commences, as it often prevents the severity of the pain. It is excellent for teenagers who are too young to go on the pill.

Heavy bleeding

Often heavy bleeding is a symptom of hormonal imbalance and therefore keeping to a healthy lifestyle is an essential part of normalizing this discomfort. You should be examined by a gynecologist to make sure you have no fibroids or other problems with your uterus.

Refer to the vital living program (see chapter 11) and see a naturopath for specific prescriptions.

❀ Use a tonic (one teaspoonful three to four times a day beginning ten days before the period) made from dong quai, shepherd's purse, cramp bark, blue cohosh, motherwort, and sage. This is a wonderful tonic that I have prescribed for many women with this problem who do not have any other problems with their hormones or uterus.

Note: Some women miss several periods during times of high stress, travel, heavy exercise, or extreme dieting. If you're not having periods and are sure you are not pregnant, try the following:

- check iron and B_{12} levels
- take one B complex tablet per day
- take evening primrose oil (3000 mg) daily
- ensure you have a regular protein intake.

Adolescent hormones

It is quite common for a young girl beginning to menstruate to have irregular cycles. A healthy diet is the key, but unfortunately it is hard to influence teenagers' eating habits; however if your teenager will follow even 70 to 80 percent of a healthy diet, supplements can be cut to a minimum. Supplements are tremendous for that extra boost of vitality and for performing well at school. Mood changes are lessened and growth patterns improve.

Try the following supplements for balanced hormones:

- Evening primrose oil capsules: two each morning.
- A complex vitamin B: one after breakfast.
- A complex mineral tablet containing calcium, magnesium, zinc, and trace minerals: one in the morning and one in the evening before bed. This last dose assists sleep and helps to strengthen bones. Calcium is laid down in the bones in adolescents between the ages of 12 to 18 and it is essential that calcium supplements (500 mg) are taken daily. I see many young girls who are dieting and will not eat dairy products.
- Iron and folic acid are vital for energy and regular cycles. For young girls who are vegetarian, an iron tablet can be beneficial. If preferred, a tonic of iron-rich herbs is also obtainable at health stores. Take one teaspoonful once to twice a day.
- Skin often tends to break out at the onset of menstruation due to the oestrogen increase. Echinacea tablets, one each morning commencing a week before periods, assist in keeping the blood cleaner and boost immunity, which is often lowered at this time.

- Even though fish oils are helpful in regulating PMT, sometimes they can aggravate breakouts in the skin. I like to increase fish in the teenager's diet with tins of salmon and fresh fish daily.
- Carrot juice, full of antioxidants, is excellent for the skin.

7

Menopause

MENOPAUSE IS A time for reflection on life and a reassessment of lifestyle. It is an exciting time and doesn't have to be painful and negative as so much of the media hype would have us believe. In fact, many women feel elated at this stage of their lives as they find that menopause represents time for them and their needs. It's a time when you can look forward to meeting new people and setting new goals, such as studying a language, or enrolling in a university course or a simple cooking course. Set goals to be healthier and wiser, and you'll be amazed at how your body will feel better. Use prescription medication sparingly, only if you need it and only when you have tried all other avenues.

Pre-menopause

Menopause, or the end of periods, usually occurs in women between the ages of 45 and 55. Menopausal symptoms can appear early, even while regular periods continue. This is often referred to as a pre-menopausal stage and can be treated very well with natural medicine. Symptoms can include anxiety, mild depression, hot flushes, urinary problems, painful intercourse, dry skin and vagina, a loss of vitality, confusion, and memory lapses.

A blood test can reveal a hormonal imbalance, although sometimes it will return a normal result even though you may be experiencing uncomfortable symptoms. Most doctors will not treat the pre-menopausal stage with hormones and will advise you to include certain foods in your diet and supplement it with natural medicine. If you experience severe depression at this stage, an antidepressant can be prescribed but I recommend you try natural therapies before resorting to strong medication. I have seen vitamin and herbal supplementation work very well in pre-menopausal women combined with regular exercise and a healthy diet.

Periods stop due to the loss of ovary function and a decline of oestrogen and progesterone. When this actually happens and you have had no periods for six months, symptoms can become more intense, although this is certainly not the case for all women. Even after periods stop, the body continues to make some small amounts of hormones from the adrenal glands while it is adjusting to the chemical changes. Women can do so many things to help themselves feel more balanced and healthier, allowing this transition stage to be easier and eliminating much of the negativity that often surrounds hormonal changes.

Pre-menopausal treatment

Refer to the dietary advice for hormones on pages 76–78 and include the following:

❀ All foods with a soya bean base have been shown to assist hot flushes and other mild menopausal symptoms. Include soya milk daily and soya beans in salads, or you can buy a soya bean powder, which is often called isoflavone powder, as this is the active ingredient in soya that assists menopausal symptoms. Take one to two teaspoonfuls per day.

❧ Add flaxseed oil to your diet as this seed contains high levels of substances known as lignan phytoestrogens, soluble fiber, and linoleic acid which helps omega–3 and –6 oils (the good fatty acids) to protect against heart disease.

❧ Drink two to three cups of sage tea per day. Traditionally this tea is well known to lift the spirit.

❧ Take a vitamin E tablet (250–500 IU) daily to act as an antioxidant and assist in counteracting heart disease and dry skin.

❧ Omega–3 and –6 through evening primrose oil and salmon oil: one capsule of each twice daily. A fish oil capsule and an evening primrose oil capsule will also assist with joint pain and insomnia.

❧ Black cohosh: one to two tablets daily or as prescribed by your naturopath or doctor if you are having mood swings or feeling down in the dumps.

- Take one B complex tablet containing 50 mg each of the Bs.

- Vitamin C is helpful for hot flushes. Also, drink and eat citrus fruits daily.

- One 1000 mg calcium supplement daily helps keep bones strong.

- Add magnesium (500 mg) to alleviate stress, and assist with muscle relaxation and calcium absorption.

- If you have hot flushes and are feeling anxious with a little depression but don't like swallowing tablets, a tonic made from equal parts of black cohosh, licorice, chasteberry, motherwort, chamomile, wild yam, and sage is excellent. Take one teaspoonful two to three times a day to relieve many of the uncomfortable pre-menopausal symptoms. I have used this for many women and, combined with the omega–3 and –6 oils, they often do not need any other vitamins (especially if they stick to the vital living program and do some exercise).

Libido

Libido is governed by well-balanced hormones and a healthy diet.
Of course, a happy relationship is also important, as is managing
stress in your life. Testosterone is a hormone that is generally
only associated with men, but many women are unaware that
they have small amounts of this hormone too. Some women do
not produce enough testosterone, which directly affects the
libido, during and after menopause. I think it's wise for a woman
to follow a healthy diet, take regular exercise, and add herbal
supplements to her regime before taking any artificial hormones.
If you have tried all avenues and have had no success after six
months, then discuss the problem with your doctor or
naturopath. Doctors often advise women who complain of low
libido to take small amounts of chemical testosterone to assist in
this problem.

Treatment

🌿 *Tribulus terrestris* is a herb that has been shown to enhance
testosterone production. This herb can also be used in

males. Combined with withania (see below), it can enhance menopausal libido. Take one tablet of each, once or twice a day or as prescribed by your naturopath. Do not take these herbs if you are experiencing PMT as they will tend to aggravate symptoms.

❀ It is important to note here that menopausal women do not produce progesterone from the ovaries but from the adrenal glands in very small amounts. Withania is therefore an important herb when women have "adrenal burn out" (see below) and temporary loss of libido from anxiety and exhaustion.

Withania
Withania helps the female body adapt to stress by enabling the adrenal glands to release adrenaline slowly and therefore allowing more consistent energy. When you are under high stress over a long time (such as from the loss of a loved one, divorce, trauma, or excessive work load) your adrenal gland

runs at an abnormally fast pace causing "adrenal burn out." Since the balance between progesterone, oestrogen and testosterone is all important for a healthy libido, this herb plays an important role for a pre- and post-menopausal woman.

Menopause

Women should be very aware of the state of their health as they approach menopause. When your periods stop completely, your doctor should arrange a bone scan to measure your bone density. You should also have a cholesterol test and a cardiovascular check, including a blood pressure reading. If you have a history of breast cancer in the family, it is usually advised not to take any forms of hormone replacement therapy (HRT) for the symptoms of menopause. That's when patients often come to me for help in relieving symptoms.

If you eat well and follow the vital living program (see chapter 11), you may sail through menopause without needing any supplementation at all.

Environmental oestrogens

Environmental oestrogens are found in meats and dairy foods, and are leached from plastics and some chemicals, especially pesticides. Exposure to these oestrogens means an increased risk of oestrogen-dependent tumors. It is important to note here that plant oestrogens in soya products (see page 99) inhibit the damaging effect of environmental oestrogens. In understanding this important action, it is vital that soya bean products are incorporated into your diet daily.

HRT or not?

Natural medicine can be beneficial on its own or in conjunction with prescribed medicines. You can only decide whether to take HRT or not when you have all the facts. The first consideration is your general health. If there is no breast cancer or osteoporosis in your family history and you have a strong cardiovascular system, you may not wish to take HRT. Similarly, if a woman has osteoporosis or if there's a family history of heart disease or breast cancer, it might be preferable to try natural medicine instead of HRT. However, if the symptoms are severe and natural medicine is not working strongly enough, HRT can be a great relief.

Bone density is a critical issue when a woman goes through menopause. In my experience, women do very well without HRT if they eat well, exercise and do weight-bearing exercises for healthy bones. If you are having bone loss even on natural medicine, then HRT should be considered. Your doctor can check your bone density every five years.

Most importantly, you should explore all options and be monitored by a naturopath and doctor to ensure that you have the best treatment for you. This way you will receive the best of both worlds.

Menopause treatment without HRT

In general, follow the dietary treatment program on pages 76–78 and the supplements recommended for the pre-menopausal program (see pages 90–92).

❧ Black cohosh: take one tablet two to three times a day.

* For insomnia take one 3 mg tablet of melatonin before bed. Menopausal women have been found to have low levels of this hormone which is vital for deep sleep and has recently been found to have anti-cancer effects.

* For depression take two to three St John's wort tablets per day and a magnesium tablet of 500 mg two to three times a day.

* A homeopathic medicine called Sepia is excellent if you are feeling lackluster and listless. Take twice a day until you are feeling better.

* For very dry skin include evening primrose oil and salmon oil capsules. I recommend one capsule of each three times a day.

* Incorporate soya products—soya milk, beans, tofu—in your daily diet.

Good foods for menopause

Soya beans: add these beans to salads and casseroles. They must be soaked overnight, then rinsed with fresh water and simmered for 45 to 60 minutes. Soya beans must be well cooked otherwise they will cause flatulence. The end product is pleasantly soft and has a nutty flavor.

Soya bean sprouts: use generously in salads and sandwiches.

Soya milk: use daily on cereals, as a drink or even in a cappuccino.

Soya flakes: can be used in porridge and as a thickener for sauces.

Soya flours: can be used in making pancakes, breads, low-fat and low-sugar cakes or cookies.

Tofu and tempeh (a form of processed soya beans): can be used in stirfried meals or mashed into rissoles with vegetables.

Miso and soya sauces (salt reduced): these sauces are used mainly for taste.

Other foods and herbs that should be included in your diet:

- Alfalfa (use sprouts in salads).
- Aniseed: use in cooking or teas. Found in the spirits Pernod and Ouzo.
- Black cohosh.

- Dong quai (a Chinese herb that is often in herbal formulas or can be prescribed by itself if black cohosh is not working for you).
- An occasional beer is okay!
- Linseed.
- Licorice (pure not commercial).
- Parsley.
- Red clover (often prescribed in the form of tablets or across the counter in the form of Promensil). It has assisted some women greatly with hot flushes and skin irritations.

Post-menopause

Menopause can last for six months or two to three years. Generally you know when it is finished when you feel back to your old self: no more hot flushes, no unusual anxiety, your hope in life is restored, and you have a positive outlook. When patients feel an improvement, I advise them to stay on their vitamins, cutting down their dosages as they feel better. If symptoms return, I advise them to go back to their former vitamin and herbal program.

Treatment to be continued post-menopause

🦋 Antioxidant tablets: one or two a day for continued well being and to act as an anti-cancer treatment.

🦋 Vitamin E: (250 or 500 IU) daily.

🦋 Fish oil for keeping cholesterol under control: two per day.

🦋 Calcium: 500 mg per day with 200 mg of magnesium.

🦋 60 mg co-enzyme Q10 tablet to restore energy and heart integrity.

🦋 If your memory is failing, take a ginkgo tablet once or twice a day, but not in the evenings as it will keep you awake.

8

Beating jet lag

IT IS ALWAYS best to prepare your body for the onslaught of jet lag when a large trip is coming up. I recommend the following program four to seven days prior to travelling.

- No alcohol.

- No refined sugar or chemicals, so no junk food or carbonated drinks.

- No caffeine in coffee or chocolate. Black tea is okay if you only drink a few cups a day.

- Eight hours sleep for at least three nights before you travel.

🌸 Take one melatonin tablet of 1–3 mg two to three nights before you travel to give you refreshed sleep and to prepare your body for a different time clock.

🌸 Keep stress levels to a minimum.

🌸 Don't miss your exercise or yoga classes beforehand just because you are busy. It is vital that your circulation is moving well before the plane trip.

🌸 If you have no exercise program, walk each day for a week prior to the journey and stretch for ten minutes twice a day to get the blood circulating around the body.

🌸 Keep your blood thin in case of blood clots on the plane by taking these supplements for a week prior to flying:
  - Evening primrose oil: one capsule after each meal.
  - Vitamin E: 200 IU once a day.
  - B_6: 100 mg once a day if you suffer from fluid retention.
  - Hawthorn berry: one capsule after each meal if you have a tendency to blood clotting or varicose veins.
  - Vitamin C with bioflavonoids: one tablet four times a

day, especially if you have a tendency to have sinus or ear problems on the plane.

On the plane

🌸 Do not eat junk food. Pre-order vegetarian meals or fruits as they are lighter on the digestion.

🌸 Drink copious amounts of water to prevent dehydration.

🌸 Try not to consume any alcohol as it is so dehydrating but, if you must, stick to a spirit mixed with soda or tonic and drink two glasses of water for every one glass of alcohol.

🌸 Move around for circulation and make sure you do the foot exercises when sitting as encouraged by the airlines to prevent any blood clots.

Treatment for jet lag

If you are going straight to bed when you arrive at your destination, follow these steps.

- Take a long, hot bath preferably with a cup of Epsom salts, which help you to sleep.

- Stretch for ten minutes.

- Take a melatonin tablet (not more than 3 mg) ten minutes before bed. Continue one tablet a day for at least three to four days to assist the body to adjust its time clock. You may take it for longer if you like.

- For those who do not like taking melatonin, take two valerian tablets to assist sleep and one calcium tablet (500–1000 mg).

- Drink a cup of loose leaf organic chamomile tea.

- If you haven't eaten properly on the plane and are hungry, have a simple vegetable soup (no spices). Avoid bread, cheese, black tea, coffee, or green tea as they tend to keep the body awake.

🌸 Do not watch violent television or the news. You may wish to watch TV to help you relax but choose a gentle program or some sleepy classical music.

Supplements

These keep the energy up and the immune system healthy as well as assisting in the relief of jet lag.

🌸 One antioxidant tablet per day.

🌸 One tablet of either echinacea, andrographis, and astragalus or cats claw or a combination tablet per day.

🌸 Two evening primrose oil capsules per day if your skin is dry and you are travelling into winter.

❧ One to two magnesium tablets per day if you are walking a lot, sightseeing, or skiing. It assists the muscles and prevents cramping.

❧ One multivitamin tablet per day that contains B, iron, and folic acid for energy and to make up for any depletions while travelling.

You may double the dosage of supplements for a few days if you are very tired or suffering from a cold, flu or virus. In this case, also add vitamin C (1000 mg) three times a day.

For women who bloat on planes and/or suffer from bowel problems and irregularity, one acidophilus capsule after each meal is a must. Otherwise eat a yogurt daily.

In-flight tips

❧ If you suffer from sinus, ask the flight attendant for the eucalyptus and peppermint inhalants that they usually have on the plane to help your respiratory system, especially when landing.

❧ You can take along a Vicks inhalant and use it to help equalize the pressure in your airways, and so prevent pain and ear problems.

❧ A homeopathic preparation called Hepar Sulph is excellent to unblock runny noses and help with allergies and sinus when flying. Take five drops under the tongue every two hours or as required.

❧ Try to sleep on the plane with a tablet of melatonin or a herbal combination of valerian, passionflower, calcium, and vervain.

❧ Wear no make-up when flying to allow your skin to breathe and use a rich night moisturizer to prevent the skin drying out. Don't forget your hands, too.

❧ Take as little as possible on the plane with you. Remember you have to carry it and with jet lag it only adds to the fatigue and frustration.

❧ Make sure you take a good book that you have started to read before the trip and can't put down. So many people quickly buy a new book at airports and don't like what they have bought.

❧ Just relax and enjoy the trip whether it is for business or a holiday.

9

Aging gracefully

IT IS COMMON knowledge that we are now living longer. Advances in medical science and surgical techniques have played their part in increasing our life spans. But one of the most important factors is that we have become much more educated about preventative medicine. We look seriously at how exercise, low-fat diets, diabetic health, eating habits, smoking, and alcohol affect us and the way we age. On top of that, there are a variety of stimulating work opportunities that were not available 50 years ago, especially for women, that keep our minds active. Scientific research is facing a huge challenge at present about the morality of extending life expectancy through the possibilities of changing the DNA of the cell. This could give us years of extra life; we could live to 150 in the next 30 years and longer by the next century.

This all sounds so overwhelming and yet the essence of living longer is all to do with our quality of life. Are we happy? Do we enjoy good health? Are we active? Are we using our brains to our full potential? Are we in happy relationships? Are we living in a stimulating environment? Dr David Weeks and Jamie Jones, who researched and wrote a book called *The Super Young*, found in summary three points that made people appear younger than their counterparts at the same age.

- These people firstly had **more energy** from being good sleepers. We certainly know scientifically that during sleep the body repairs the brain, restores depleted substances, and repairs damaged cell tissue.
- Secondly, these people had a **stronger resilience** to the stresses of life and had the ability to "bounce back" from disasters in their lives.
- Thirdly, they had the **capacity to adapt** to new situations or anything a little unfamiliar.

Preventing aging

The qualities of energy, resilience, and adaptability are not, as this study found, all genetic. People *work* on their health to have more energy. And taking supplementary vitamins and foods increases circulation to the brain to give greater "brain power." The following can be incorporated in your daily living to obtain, over a period of time, greater energy and sharper mental facilities.

- Follow a three-day detox program of raw vegetable and fruit juices and vegetable soups. This will lay the foundation of better health and clean out pollutants in your system.

- Include antioxidant foods in your diet and eat fresh vegetables and fruits daily.

- Low blood sugar levels interfere with proper brain function, as the brain needs fuel. Therefore eat three meals a day and protein snacks or fruit in between meals if you suffer from low blood sugar.

❧ Eat quality protein to regenerate cell tissue—cold-water fish, legumes such as soya beans, chickpeas, lentils and haricot beans, eggs, nuts, low-fat cheese, free-range chicken, and a little red meat if you are not vegetarian.

❧ Cut out 80 percent of your junk foods, including carbonated drinks, refined sugars, processed meats, and tinned foods, and cut down alcohol consumption (this is also proven to destroy brain cells in excess).

❧ Drink eight glasses of fresh filtered water daily and include herbal teas to your taste.

❧ Drink raw juices as they contain enzymes for cell rejuvenation.

❧ Drink some form of concentrated green juice such as wheat grass juice (one tablespoonful a day mixed with carrot juice or water), or spirulina or green barley juice. They are rich in peptides and enzymes, which are essential for the development of the feel good hormones such as endorphins.

❧ Exercise regularly (three times a week or more).

❧ Stretch or do yoga to keep your joints and muscles supple.

❧ Spend time outdoors in fresh air with trees or water or mountains.

❧ Keep out of the strong rays of the midday sun (they can be cancer-forming and aging).

❧ Keep stress levels down as stress depletes important minerals and vitamin B.

❧ Find a happy work environment.

❧ Do all you can to get out of an unhappy relationship, even if this means you will be on a lower income.

❧ Enjoy friends of all ages and make it your business to be involved with younger people.

🦋 Stop smoking and taking recreational drugs as it is proven that they are detrimental to your brain faculties and destroy brain cells.

Preventative vitamins and herbs

🦋 One antioxidant tablet per day.

🦋 One to two ginkgo tablets per day (not at night as it will keep you awake).

🦋 One vitamin E per day (300–500 IU if you do not have high blood pressure, otherwise check the dosage with your doctor).

🦋 One co-enzyme Q10 per day of 60–100 mg.

🦋 Selenium: 20–30 mg per day.

❧ One or two 500 mg magnesium tablets per day to assist in calming the brain and reducing anxiety as these symptoms interfere in concentration and learning ability.

❧ One to two fish oil capsules per day with omega–3 and –6 for the lubrication of joints and prevention of myelin sheath wear and tear (see pages 118–119).

❧ Lecithin: 2000 mg per day as it contains choline, which protects and restores dendrites in the brain, essential for memory and sharp thinking. It was found in one study that patients with memory loss experienced up to 50 percent improvement just from choline supplementation. Foods high in lecithin are egg yolks, soya beans, wheat germ, and whole wheat products.

❧ Melatonin: one 1–3 mg tablet when sleeping is poor.

❧ Vitamin B complex (B_5 is important): 50–100 mg three times a day.

Antioxidants

We hear about antioxidants through the media and in health books but very few people really know what the word antioxidant means or how they work. "Anti" means "against." Oxidation is a process that begins at birth when oxygen is taken into the body and begins life but also begins death since oxygen breaks down tissue. The best example is when you cut an apple in two. After a few minutes it begins to turn brown. Oxidation is setting in. To delay this we keep fruit and vegetables in the fridge. Organic grains and teas should also be placed in the fridge to slow down oxidation.

Researchers have discovered that certain substances called free radicals (the nasties) are formed just through living. Free radicals have the ability to break down healthy tissue, which leads to cancers, heart disease, chronic bowel problems, and numerous other illnesses prevalent in the twenty-first century. We are aware now that major factors in our modern lifestyle have a profound effect on free radical production, including pollution, refined fatty foods, stress, smoking, recreational drugs, and viruses.

By taking antioxidants regularly through food and vitamins we are slowing down free radical damage. Antioxidants are an essential part of daily living and not only increase our life span but also increase the quality of our life through greater well being and vitality. The main foods that have concentrates of antioxidants are all orange fruits and vegetables such as oranges, sweet potato, pumpkin, carrots, mangoes, peaches, pawpaw, nectarines, and apricots. They contain vitamins C and A. Vitamin E, found in avocados, wheatgerm oils, and in smaller amounts in cold-pressed olive oils and cold-pressed vegetable oils, is also a vital antioxidant. Certain herbs and other food substances have been found to have significant antioxidant properties. They are garlic, sage, turmeric, rosemary, shisandra, and St Mary's thistle, green tea and black tea, grape seed, and co-enzyme Q10.

Fish oils

Fish oils have been found to protect the myelin sheath, which is to the nerves like the outer plastic coat of an electrical wire. Myelin acts as an insulator and protects the sensitive nerves helping to conduct impulses. It is thought that those who have keen mental powers into later age may have a genetic predisposition that protects the myelin sheath from breaking down. All of us are wise to take fish oils, ginkgo, and antioxidants. Multiple sclerosis sufferers have been found to have inflammation of the myelin sheath and research is holding out positive hope for more findings on how to restore this sheath in the chronic stages of this illness.

Ginkgo (*ginkgo biloba*)

The ginkgo is a deciduous tree that has been around for 150 million years. The research of German scientists in the 1960s showed that ginkgo is an excellent treatment for circulation problems. The herb brings more oxygen to the tissues, particularly brain tissue. The leaves contain active substances known as flavonoids. Ginkgo is wonderful for treating problems of memory, tinnitus, dizziness, and the effects of high altitude. It is especially helpful for the early effects of dementia. I use it frequently to enhance memory, particularly in the 50-plus age group.

Stress

High levels of continued stress produce an overabundance of a hormone from the adrenal glands called cortisol. The part of the brain that shuts off this production deteriorates with age. When this happens the person reacts even more strongly to stress and can suffer even more damage to the "shut off" mechanism. Research has found that stress is magnified when people feel out of control. Also, it has been discovered that if you are to reduce your stress levels, holding in the problem must be avoided, so it is good to chat to a friend or family member or see a counselor.

Brain power

Alertness and memory are key issues for the modern woman who wishes to age gracefully. It's important to keep up any hobby that uses the brain. Remember the brain is an organ that must be exercised daily. Take on new challenges with study, languages, reading, and mind games, such as any form of puzzles using numbers, words, or sentences.

Brain cells do not regenerate, therefore it is vital to preserve what you have and assist your memory powers with natural medicines. Scientists have found that three main factors affect longevity and the potential onset of dementia:

- raised homocystine levels in the blood (this can be tested by your doctor);
- poor circulation and atherosclerosis (hardening of the arteries);
- inflammation (from arthritis, coeliac disease, irritable bowel, allergies, toxic exposure, alcohol, smoking).

Treatment

❧ B_{12} and folic acid: 300–400 mg of each lowers homocystine levels with B_6, 100 mg daily.

❧ Herbs such as ginkgo and Bacopa are vital for circulation to the brain.

❧ An antioxidant tablet with vitamins E, C, and A plus herbs from your naturopath can be of great assistance to stop the effects of free radical damage—hardening of the arteries and other tissue damage which causes inflammation of various parts of the body.

Schisandra
(*Schisandra chinensis*)

In the Chinese medical system, schisandra is regarded as one of the great antioxidant herbs with an amazing ability to detoxify the liver and to relieve mental fatigue.

10

Common female ailments

OFTEN RECURRING minor ailments indicate an imbalance in eating habits. These symptoms can range from thrush to weak nails to a bloated stomach. When you change your diet by adopting the vital living program (see chapter 11), you'll find that most of these minor issues begin to clear. If you are continually experiencing symptoms that are not related to a more serious condition, it can often be your body telling you that you need to slow down and attend to the problem before it turns into a larger one.

Sometimes minor symptoms can be hereditary, but there is always a natural way of remedying them before resorting to medication. Preventative action is the key factor here.

Headaches

These can be a sign of any of the following:

- Hormonal imbalance
- A vertebra problem in the neck
- A muscle tightness in the neck or back
- Gallstones and kidney stones
- Constipation
- Stress
- Low blood sugar levels.

It is important that you address the problem that is the most likely cause of your discomfort. You will find treatments for many of the above conditions outlined in this book. Turn to the appropriate chapter and follow the program outlined. Monitor any progress. Another way to reduce headaches is to begin the vital living program (see chapter 11) by eliminating junk food, eating more healthily, and exercising regularly. If you have back problems, swimming is the finest exercise.

Treatment

❄ For any form of headaches I will always prescribe magnesium in powder form or tablet, 400–600 mg daily, as this mineral is marvellous to relax muscle tissue and relieve spasms.

❄ If there is inflammation from an injury, then an antioxidant tablet three times a day is essential with one tablet of bioflavonoids three times a day.

❄ Some of my clients obtain a lot of relief from a herb called feverfew, one tablet three times a day. In traditional herbal medicine this herb was always used as a preventative and a cure for migraine headaches.

Nausea

This can be a sign of several things:
- Pregnancy
- Gall bladder problems

- Overloaded stomach
- Poor digestion.

Treatment

❧ Ginger tablets are marvellous for all of the above and very safe to use during pregnancy. Take one capsule after every meal. If gallstones run in the family, ask your doctor for an ultrasound.

❧ Take one fish oil capsule after each meal or evening primrose oil if fish oil does not agree with you in smell or taste. These oils assist the gall bladder to eliminate bile, which in turn helps to break down fatty foods in the digestive tract.

Cystitis

Mild cystitis is recognized by a feeling of discomfort around the bladder area and the need to urinate frequently. In the severe stages cystitis becomes an infection in the bladder and you can experience a burning feeling during urination. Before resorting to antibiotics, try natural medicine, which is often very successful. Regular preventative work is essential if you have been suffering these symptoms for a while.

Preventative program

* Not drinking water regularly can cause cystitis, so drink eight to ten glasses a day.

* Cranberry juice, one to two glasses a day, has been found to help a great deal as it has the ability to slough off the nasty bacteria that cling to the walls of the urinary tract.

* Daily garlic intake can also assist. If you prefer tablets, take one per day and have a fresh clove every second day.

Treatment

- A glass of water every hour.

- Two to three glasses of cranberry juice daily (although this is more of a preventative measure).

- Make some barley water. Use 1 cup of barley to 1 litre of water and simmer for 20 minutes. Strain and drink the water with the juice of a quarter of a lemon in each glass. Barley water is wonderful to soothe irritated bladder walls and flush out any residual infection.

- Echinacea tablets or liquid assist in fighting the infection. Take one tablet every four hours or a teaspoonful of the tincture every four hours.

- Non-acidic vitamin C (such as Ester C): a teaspoonful in water every four hours.

- Garlic tablets: one every four hours.

❦ When the symptoms are better (after 36 hours), continue to use the supplements three times a day for two weeks.

If the cystitis does not improve then you may need an antibiotic. You may still run the natural medicines alongside this, as it will help your natural immune system. Be aware that cystitis can be an ongoing problem if you do not drink at least eight glasses of water daily.

Thrush

Thrush shows itself with an annoying white discharge from the vagina that can cause itching. Sometimes thrush can show in the mouth as a white filmy residue on the tongue. It can be exacerbated before and during your period. Thrush is a sign of *Candida albicans*, an overgrowth of the bacterium candida, and often occurs when an overuse of antibiotics wipes out much of the bowel's healthy bacteria. Hence eat plenty of yogurt with acidophilus when taking antibiotics and avoid foods high in sugar, as sugar feeds candida.

Preventative program

🍀 Stop eating foods that encourage candida, such as yeasty foods like bread, wine, beer, and fermented cheeses, and refined sugars such as chocolates, sugary desserts, cakes, and sweets.

🍀 Eat a yogurt daily with added acidophilus, include garlic in your food as much as possible, and make sure you are not constipated as this breeds more of the candida.

Treatment

🍀 Take half a teaspoonful of acidophilus powder (available at health stores) in a glass of water before breakfast and dinner.

🍀 Combine half a teaspoonful of the powder with a little water to make a paste in your hand and place into your vagina two to three times a day.

❀ You may use the acidophilus powder in a douche with four drops of golden seal and four drops of calendula and two drops of tea-tree oil. Do not put straight tea-tree oil into the vagina, as it is too strong.

❀ There are pessaries made from similar herbs that can be used internally twice a day until the discharge clears. These are obtainable at a health store.

❀ Garlic has been found to help eliminate thrush through its antibacterial affect. Take a tablet after each meal until better.

It is important to note that any bacteria from a bowel motion needs to be wiped away thoroughly from the area between the vagina and the anus.

Vaginal dryness

This condition can be treated with a cream made from a base of vitamin E with 10 ml of calendual oil, 10 ml of evening primrose oil and 20 ml of olive oil. This can be applied morning and evening.

Fibroids and cysts

Fibroids in the uterus or on the ovaries are quite common with many women. They can occur in women of all ages and an ultrasound will establish how big they are. Prolonged pain and discomfort in the pelvic area and acne are some symptoms that may indicate you have fibroids or cysts. Check with your doctor to ascertain if they are any threat to your ongoing health. Sometimes they need to be removed surgically if they are large. Generally women feel much better after this procedure, especially without the continual bloating that accompanies fibroids.

Often smaller cysts come and go on the ovaries according to a woman's cycle. Women are often given the contraceptive pill to assist in regulating oestrogen and progesterone and this will reduce the occurrence of cysts.

Treatment

❧ B$_6$: 200 mg daily helps to dispel minor cysts.

❧ Magnesium can assist in pain: 100 mg two to three times per day.

❧ Chasteberry: one tablet a day for two weeks before your period often takes away many of the minor symptoms and is safe and effective even for adolescents.

Healthy hearts and veins

Hereditary patterns play a major role in problems related to the heart and circulation. However, the following preventative and treatment programs are vital for those that have a tendency toward high cholesterol and blood pressure. They are even more essential for those who do not exercise and who smoke, are overweight, have a high alcohol intake and eat junk food high in fat and refined products. From a naturopathic perspective, women who have followed a low-fat diet and included soya beans

and greens in their daily diet have lower incidences of heart
disease and cholesterol.

Preventative program

* Avoid deep-fried foods completely and cut right back on
  saturated fat, which includes butter, high-fat milk and
  cream, and cheese. Use low-fat substitutes.

* Sauté foods in olive oil or vegetable oil only once a week.
  It's much better to grill, steam, and bake (without fat or
  oil).

* Cut right back on chocolate. Use carob or freshly stewed
  fruits in season or a muesli bar with grains and dried
  fruit.

* Be careful of eating too many nuts such as brazil,
  peanuts, and macadamias. Cut back and eat only a small
  handful of almonds once or twice a week.

❀ Drink lots of freshly squeezed citrus fruits such as oranges, pineapples, and lemons as they are helpful in cutting back cholesterol.

❀ Include avocados and salmon for their omega–3 and –6 to assist the "good" form of cholesterol. Use cold-pressed oils on salads, but do not use any oil if you have high to very high cholesterol.

❀ Exercise regularly with some cardio or aerobic work. Ask at your gym for help determining the level you should be working at and what your heart rate should be. Power walking daily for an hour before or after work (or during the day for a mother) is ideal. Then you can take the weekend off.

❀ Stretch your muscles so your blood can eliminate any fluid gathering in the lower part of your body. Yoga or pilates is good for this.

❀ Keep the circulation moving by drinking fresh filtered water in between meals (approximately 1–2 liters a day).

🌿 Every month do a three-day detox.

🌿 Include garlic three times a week.

Treatment for cholesterol

Many women have high cholesterol when they are going through a hormonal change and this should be addressed. Check with your doctor to determine your ratio of good and bad cholesterol. You need to fast for eight hours before this blood test for a correct reading.

🌿 Follow the preventative program on pages 134–136.

🌿 Take salmon oil capsules, one tablet three to four times per day.

🌿 Vitamin E: 500 IU per day

🌿 Take a herbal capsule made from St Mary's thistle, dandelion, and schisandra (this is wonderful to detoxify the liver, which is involved in making cholesterol).

❧ Include globe artichokes when possible in your diet.

❧ Use dandelion coffee instead of normal coffee. Roasted dandelion root is delicious as a coffee substitute.

❧ Drink a glass of water each morning with the juice of a lemon to detoxify the liver before the day begins.

❧ Drink filtered water during the day and herb tea such as hawthorn berry tea or dandelion tea.

❧ Cut back on alcohol and try to drink red wine only—one or two glasses three times a week.

❧ Garlic capsules reduce fatty deposits. Take one clove a day or garlic tablets with allicin, two to three per day.

Treatment for high blood pressure

If you follow the advice given above you will lose weight, which is a must for anyone overweight with cardiovascular problems. The following supplements and guidelines are beneficial for those with high blood pressure.

🌿 Low dose vitamin E: 100–200 IU daily (check with your doctor).

🌿 No caffeine in tea, coffee, or green tea, as caffeine raises blood pressure.

🌿 An antioxidant tablet with vitamins A, C, and E (check again with doctor) daily.

🌿 A co-enzyme Q10 tablet: 30–60 mg per day, as this is vital for any heart problem.

🌿 Fish oil capsules: one after breakfast and one after dinner.

🌿 Meditation assists in bringing down blood pressure.

🌿 A herb called hawthorn berry is wonderful to assist normal heart function and can be taken whether you have high or low blood pressure. It also helps fluid retention around the ankles. Take one tablet three times per day after each meal.

🌸 Garlic tablets: one at night and one in the morning. Garlic has been shown to reduce blood pressure.

🌸 Reduce stress levels (see chapter 3).

Pain and palpitations

Some women experience pains in the chest, which they ignore. Check it out. You could be experiencing some form of angina, especially if you are in the 50-plus age bracket.

Heart palpitations are also common. If your heart is in good working order include 300–500 mg (powder or tablet) of magnesium a day. Magnesium is marvellous for regulating the rhythm of the heart and can be used by anyone, regardless of age. If palpitations are serious see a doctor. Magnesium can be safely used for panic attacks too (see page 53).

Varicose veins

Salt injections can treat fine broken capillaries but the following program may clear the veins and prevent broken capillaries from occurring further.

- One bioflavonoid tablet of 500 mg with 1000–2000 mg of vitamin C for absorption, three times a day. They are wonderful to strengthen the fine vein walls.

- Include freshly squeezed orange juice with all the pithy part that contains the bioflavonoids in your diet. Pineapple juice and fruits rich in vitamin A, such as mangoes, apricots, peaches, and papaya, all strengthen vein walls.

- Horse chestnut herb is useful for all varicose veins: one tablet after each meal.

- Vitamin E: 200–600 IU daily. This vitamin is the number-one antioxidant for veins.

❧ Calcium: 500 mg a day. This known to strengthen vein walls.

❧ Sleep with a pillow under your feet to assist blood flow and keep your feet up as often as possible.

❧ A tablet made from grapeseed extract is also excellent for the veins (and skin). Take one tablet twice per day.

Horse chestnut (*Aesculus hippocastanum*)

This is a wonderful herb for varicose veins especially if there is oedema (swelling) of the feet or legs. It doesn't help fine broken capillaries on the face. Horse chestnut works very well in elderly patients and if you are prone to thrombosis after surgery. It can also be used as a preventative for blood clotting when flying. One to three 200 mg tablets of a 5:1 concentrate recommended per day.

🌿 Use a calendula cream mixed with echinacea and witchhazel and rub into the veins daily, especially if you have some eczema in the area.

🌿 If you do not have high blood pressure, ginkgo is effective for circulation. Take one tablet twice per day, but at least four hours before you go to bed, as it tends to stimulate the brain and keep you awake.

Healthy kidneys

Our kidneys are very precious. There are only two of them and they are vital for excreting wastes and reabsorbing any trace minerals and other elements that can be useful. Kidneys have millions of fine tubules like a very complicated plumbing system. It is vital for good health that we keep this tubing clean and drained by taking in fresh liquids daily. If this is not done, stagnant wastes accumulate in these tubes causing blockages, which can lead to infections such as cystitis, kidney stones, and fluid retention.

Maintenance program

Ingesting quality liquids is most important for healthy kidneys.

- Drink eight to ten glasses of filtered water daily, and during and after exercise to clear the accumulation of wastes and toxins that are released.

- Begin the day with a glass of water at room temperature with the juice of half a lemon.

- Include a glass of freshly squeezed orange, mango, or watermelon juice in your daily intake.

- Include a raw juice of an orange and green vegetable daily. Try carrot juice mixed with spinach, wheatgrass, and parsley or add a teaspoon of the powder of a green juice such as spirulina or green barley juice.

- Include fresh homemade soup for a meal or entrée three to four times a week. In summer these can be substituted for fresh salads.

✿ Eat two to three pieces of whole fruit daily.

✿ Cut out refined sugar in carbonated drinks, sugar in tea
  and coffee, excessive amounts of alcohol, cakes and sweet
  refined snacks, and smoking.

✿ Include a yogurt daily for the good bacteria acidophilus.

✿ Drink a preservative-free cranberry juice daily if you have
  a tendency to cystitis.

Cranberry 'Una de gato' (*Vaccinium macrocarpon*)

It is now scientifically proven that cranberry juice
contains procyanidins, which work by stopping bacteria
from clinging to the mucosal walls of the urinary tract.
For women who have had chronic urinary tract
problems, it is vital to include this juice on a regular
basis to prevent infections. Always look for the purest
form of cranberry juice as some contain added sugar.

11

Eating for health

I HAVE SET OUT a vital living program that can be used for ideas and inspiration when choosing foods and groups of foods that will give you more energy. I've focused on including plenty of antioxidant foods, such as fresh fruits and vegetables. You should also include a variety of meat and vegetarian proteins that are so needed for vitality, cell regrowth, and also for weight loss.

The vital living program can be used as a lifestyle. In fact the more you eat fresh vegetables and fruits and quality protein, the more you will steer away from refined foods. You may choose to treat a specific problem with the remedies suggested in this book before starting the vital living program. Or you may start the program right now and then when you are ready you may lead on to the chapter that addresses your individual health problems. You will find that you can then incorporate the changes in diet to suit your problems and take the appropriate supplements.

I have suggested the maximum supplement program but in my practice I have noticed that some clients cannot swallow tablets or take tonics. All is not lost. Diet is the most important foundation in all areas of becoming healthier. So just try the changes in your diet or begin the vital living program with regular exercise. When you regain more energy and routine and feel comfortable with yourself and your eating habits then try to take one or two vitamin supplements that I recommend for your problem as you will find it really does work.

If you want to detox for three days before you begin a healthier lifestyle then I would advise you to obtain my book *Detox* that will guide you through the process simply with soups, raw juices, and rest.

With the vital living program there is plenty to choose from. Remember that what you eat today is how you will feel tomorrow. By accumulating good habits, whether eating at home or out in a restaurant, you are investing in your future by preventing major debilitating diseases.

If you really want to include something naughty in your diet such as a rich dessert or chocolate or sweet things then incorporate them in moderation, such as once every fourth day, and treat yourself as a reward for being so good with your healthy foods. I always say that 90 percent good and 10 percent naughty is a fairly reasonable formula for living in the twenty-first century, with all its temptations.

Here the vital living program is essential to give you inspiration and motivation to incorporate small changes. I have used these ideas on many of my clients over the years and it is amazing how easy they find it to incorporate the program into their lifestyle without having to feel the odd person out at a dinner party or in a restaurant.

The vital living program

As soon as you wake in the morning drink a glass of fresh filtered water at room temperature, which is gentle on the digestive juices and doesn't send them into shock in the way very hot or very cold drinks would. Add the juice of half a lemon with half a teaspoonful of honey if you like.

Breakfast

🦋 A high-fiber cereal such as Weet-bix or muesli, or an oatmeal or rice porridge (these are great in winter, especially sprinkled with ground almonds for protein and wheatgerm for vitamin B). Use low-fat milk with added calcium, or a low-fat soya or rice milk for those with allergies. If preferred, you can replace milk with freshly squeezed fruit juice. Sprinkle a teaspoonful of lecithin granules over the cereal (excellent for assisting the nervous system in times of stress).

🦋 A low-fat soya or dairy milk drink with a protein powder made from soya products or whey powder. Mix two to three glasses of milk with two teaspoonfuls of protein powder and add a fruit of your choice (bananas can be fattening for those watching their weight).

🦋 Toast and protein. With one or two slices of a wholemeal or soya (grainy) toast (yeast free if necessary), have a boiled or poached egg, or avocado and tomato, or tuna or salmon with black pepper. You can vary your proteins in the morning, especially if you are trying to lose weight. Baked beans are an excellent source of protein if you are doing a lot of exercise in the mornings.

❋ A bowl of fresh fruit salad with a dairy or soya yogurt with added acidophilus. Make sure you have yogurt or a protein with the fruit. If you eat only fruit in the morning, the sugar metabolizes within an hour and you may be tempted to snack on junk food. Note: Don't eat citrus fruits with stone fruits if your stomach feels bloated.

You should include plenty of fluids in your diet. For breakfast, concentrate on fresh fruit juices.

❋ A freshly squeezed fruit juice – orange, pineapple, watermelon, mango, or dark grape juice. Have just one fruit on its own, particularly if your digestion is sensitive. Vegetable juice is not ideal first thing in the morning as it can often make you feel a little nauseous due to its liver-cleansing properties. It's better drunk later in the morning or afternoon.

🌺 If you have an acidic stomach, try a cup of black tea before breakfast, as the tannin can assist this problem.

Morning snacks

🌺 One or two pieces of fruit.

🌺 A dairy, soya or goats milk yogurt with acidophilus.

🌺 Three or four Ryevita or Vita Weat crackers or rice crackers with a protein spread, such as cottage cheese, a slice of chicken, tahini, or a small tin of tuna or salmon. These snacks are especially good for those trying to lose weight and who have a tendency to eat too much sugar in cakes, muffins, and croissants.

🌺 A small handful of nuts and dried fruits. (Do not include this snack if you are overweight.)

❧ A muesli bar.

❧ A slice of nut bread with a scraping of low-fat butter.

Yogurt

Throughout every civilization in history, people have consumed cultured milk containing the good bacteria, *Lactobacillius acidophilus*. It wasn't until the beginning of the twentieth century that a man named Elie Metchnikoff put forward his theory that the longevity of the Bulgarians was due in part to their consumption of fermented milk product called "yohourth." He believed that the *Lactobacillus bulgaricus* in the product prevented poisons putrefying in the bowel causing disease and poor absorption of nutrients. These early findings have now become scientific facts. We now know that the lactobacilli in our diet fights against not only cancer but also many other diseases.

Lunch

🌿 A sandwich of grainy or soya linseed bread or a yeast-free
bread (such as pita) with a protein—egg, chicken,
legumes, tempeh, tofu, salmon, or tuna—and a green,
orange, and white salad.

🌿 A salad with a protein, as above, and add a carbohydrate
if you like, such as brown rice, buckwheat, couscous, or
potato salad.

🌿 Rice with vegetables and fish, or tofu or a legume.

🌿 A vegetable soup with a protein such as chicken or a
legume such as kidney beans.

🌿 A pasta or noodle dish with three colored vegetables and
a vegetarian protein.

Note: If you only eat fruit salad for lunch, you will be hungry
within one to two hours as the high sugar content metabolizes
faster than proteins and grains. Make sure you eat a protein

snack as well, otherwise you will have the tendency to crave sweets, cakes, and sugary snacks in the afternoon.

Afternoon snacks

Choose an option from morning snacks (see pages 150–151).

Dinner

🌿 Grilled or steamed fish (preferably a cold-water fish such as salmon and tuna) with four colored vegetables (raw or cooked): green—spinach, lettuce, rocket, peas, brussels sprouts; orange—sweet potato, carrots, pumpkin; white—potato, cauliflower, cucumber; and red—capsicum, tomatoes.

🌿 A protein such as red meat, free-range chicken, or a legume with the vegetables described above.

🌿 Brown rice or a mixture of different rices with a protein as above. Add some lightly steamed vegetables.

* Couscous or buckwheat with vegetables and protein.

* Casseroled vegetables and a protein served on a base of rice, couscous, or buckwheat.

* Barbecued or grilled protein and vegetables with a green salad on the side.

* A thick vegetable and chicken soup with barley. Chickpeas and dried bean mix can be use instead of chicken.

* A large mixed vegetable salad with a protein such as a boiled egg, tuna, or salmon or steamed chicken or avocado. Add extra flavor with spices or fresh herbs, such as parsley, ginger, or mint.

* A pasta dish. Make sure you buy rice pasta if you are allergic to wheat. Combine with a seafood, meat, or chicken sauce. Always serve with a green salad.

Notes

Add spices, vegetable salt, mint, fresh basil, and parsley to any of your vegetables, especially if you steam them, as this is a healthy and tasty way of including more vegetables in your diet.

If you are watching your weight:

- Do not fry foods.
- Do not use sauces on your foods.
- Do not overeat at night (make sure your stomach is not bursting when you leave the table after a meal).
- Do not drink excessive alcohol while eating.
- Do not eat just before bed. Eat at least four hours before sleeping.

Dessert

❧ A bowl of fresh or stewed fruit and yogurt.

❧ Rice pudding with a small amount of sugar. This is good for those craving dessert.

🌸 Watermelon (excellent for weight watchers and it can satisfy the sweet craving at the end of a meal).

Supper

🌸 A yogurt.

🌸 A small bowl of stewed fruit.

🌸 A glass of milk, soya milk, or rice milk.

Fluid intake

🌸 Filtered water: eight glasses a day. Best drunk in between meals.

🌸 Freshly squeezed raw fruit and vegetable juice: one of each daily.

❦ Herbal tea: one cup three to four times a day. This can be counted in your water intake.

❦ Green tea: one cup twice a day. This can be counted as part of your water intake.

❦ Black tea: one cup once a day.

❦ A glass of red wine: twice a week.

This vital living program is recommended for every woman wanting to improve their energy levels and their general health. I suggest the following modifications and variations for women of different ages. If you have a specific complaint, refer to the relevant chapter in this book.

Ages 12 to 18

Teenage girls need plenty of calcium for their growing bones.

❦ Include one to two dairy products twice daily: low-fat milk, cheese and yogurt, or almonds. If you don't eat

these foods, supplement your diet with a mineral tablet
of 150 mg of calcium and 20–30 mg of magnesium.

❧ Include soya products (see page 99) to assist hormonal
balance.

❧ Eat cold-water fish three times a week. This is good for
the skin and hormonal balance, and assists concentration
at school. If you don't eat fish, supplement with one
omega–3 and –6 oil capsule twice a day.

❧ Weight-bearing exercise is essential for making strong
bones. Do some intense sport three times a week. Yoga,
dance, and walking are also good.

Ages 20 to 35

Partying and late nights can take a toll.

❧ Drink plenty of water.

❧ B vitamins are essential when drinking alcohol.

❧ Take brewer's yeast (not the same yeast as in bread) and mix a teaspoonful in a glass of water daily, otherwise make sure brown rice and wholemeal grains are eaten daily.

Ages 35 to 45

Weight can creep up on this age group.

❧ Include yogurt with acidophilus daily to assist the digestion or take an acidophilus capsule twice a day.

❧ Skin becomes drier through subtle hormonal changes. Include cold-water fish three to four times a week for the omega–3 oils and take an evening primrose oil capsule (1000 mg) twice a day or flaxseed oil (one teaspoonful) daily.

❧ Check you are not eliminating all dairy foods from your diet as you need calcium to combat the beginning of hormonal changes, which can happen as early as the forties.

Ages 45 to 55

❧ Make sure you include soya products and calcium-enriched foods daily.

❧ Eat smaller meals as your metabolism may be starting to slow down, which can cause weight problems.

❧ Eat less and exercise regularly.

Age 55 and onwards

Enjoy life. Be sensible with your vital living program.

❧ Take as few prescription medicines as possible and make a concerted effort to eat for health!

Choosing vitamins: quality and dosage

🍀 Look for organic brands wherever possible, without additives, colorings, or preservatives. Choose yeast- and sugar-free supplements. The label should state all ingredients. If not, choose a brand that does.

🍀 When buying herbal supplements (tablets or liquids), by law the standardized extract of the herb must be included on the label. For example, *Ginkgo biloba* supplements must say that they contain however many milligrams of the extract of the active ingredient. A naturopath can help you work out the individual dosages of certain brands.

🍀 Make sure any fish oils you buy are sourced from farms without chemicals and wastes from the oceans. This can be checked by ringing the supplier.

🍀 Therapeutic doses can be very different from preventative doses. A naturopath will often give you much higher doses of a vitamin as a treatment than you would give yourself following the instructions on the label. Naturopaths know the effects and can monitor you closely. Once you have improved, they will lower the dosage and it will be used as a preventative measure.

❧ If a supplement disagrees with you, check that you ingested it with food and not on an empty stomach. Cut the dosage down to half and persevere for a few days. If you still seem to have indigestion or heartburn from the tablet, see your naturopath or ring the helpline for that product.

❧ If you have known allergies, read the label to make sure there are no ingredients that are likely to react badly with you.

❧ Don't take vitamins or supplements just because they are the latest trend, or because your friends have recommended them. Read each of these chapters and see what is suitable for you.

❧ Try to use locally made brands, as you should then have a support system or inquiry centre that you can call for free information. When you call this local number, which is usually stated on the label, specially trained people should be able to give you any additional advice you need.

❧ Check use-by dates and comply with them. Do not use vitamins and herbs months after opening, as oxidation will have set in and destroyed any active substances. If you are unsure, check with your naturopath or the supplier.

❧ Never take old vitamins that you are unsure of. Take them to your local health store and ask if they are suitable for you.

❧ Always keep your supplements and liquids in a dark cupboard and out of reach of small children. Unless otherwise stated, they do not need to be refrigerated.

Acknowledgements

I would like to thank my dedicated team at Penguin for their untiring assistance with this book: Julie Gibbs, Executive Publisher; Kirsten Abbott, my editor; Catherine Hanger, who helped to write this book; and all the staff who have helped organize the endless steps in the publishing process.

I thank all the women who have filled me with awe during my professional years as a naturopath—their stories and life experiences are truly remarkable.

I thank the staff at Mediherb and Healthworld for their assistance with technical information. Their dedication to maintaining high standards of vitamins and herbs is outstanding.

I thank Denis Stewart, my teacher in herbal medicine, for his pioneering work in the field of natural medicine, and his principles and skills that I can always draw upon in my own practice.

Lastly, thank you to my friends and family for encouraging me to follow my dreams in inspiring people to a healthier way of life.

Index

PENELOPE SACH is a practitioner of naturopathic, homeopathic and herbal medicine. She has studied in China and France, and now runs a highly successful clinic in Sydney, where she specializes in treating career professionals, sportspeople, and busy homemakers whose lifestyles lead to stress and fatigue.

Penelope has developed a range of organically grown herbal teas that sells widely across Australia and Asia. Her most recent book was *Detox*.

For more about Penelope Sach,
visit www.penelopesach.com.au